NUTRITION
AND
ATHLETIC
PERFORMANCE

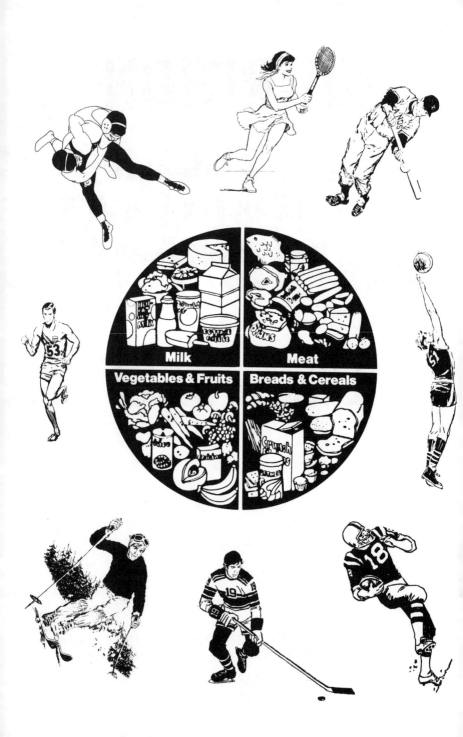

NUTRITION
AND
ATHLETIC
PERFORMANCE

Ellington Darden

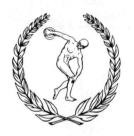

THE ATHLETIC PRESS
P.O. Box 2314-D
Pasadena, California 91105

NUTRITION AND ATHLETIC PERFORMANCE

Copyright © 1976 by Ellington Darden
All Rights Reserved
Published by The Athletic Press
Pasadena, California 91105 U.S.A.

Library of Congress Catalog Card No. 76-10811
I.S.B.N. 0-87095-058-4

1st Printing - June 1976
2nd Printing - November 1976
3rd Printing - March 1977
4th Printing - August 1977
5th Printing - January 1978
6th Printing - December 1978
7th Printing - September 1981

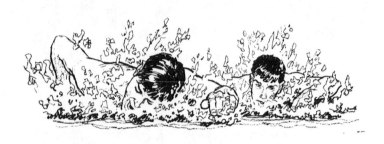

Library of Congress Cataloging in Publication Data

Darden, Ellington, 1943-
  Nutrition and athletic performance.

  Bibliography: p.
  Includes index.
  1. Athletes--Nutrition. I. Title.
TX361.A8D37   613.2'02'4796   76-10811
ISBN 0-87095-058-4

COVER PHOTOGRAPH by Ken Neely

Foreword

MANY OF OUR sports programs today are vigorous and combative, frequently involving body contact. Injuries can and do occur to all parts of the body, from head to toe and from the most superficial layers of the skin to the innermost organs of the body.

All too often coaches, trainers, and athletes themselves devote many hours to methods and techniques to improve physical performance, but neglect one of the most important components of physical readiness — optimum nutrition.

We are what we eat, and if our athletes are to have maximum performance and protection from injury, then they must have optimum nutrition.

Nutrition is important in helping to promote physical readiness and injury prevention, and also is essential in promoting rapid healing and recovery following injury and illness.

One of the most notable differences between athletes and non-athletes with similar injuries is the desire to return to competition in the shortest possible time. Without proper nutrition, this goal for the athlete will not be readily attained.

Dr. Ellington Darden, a former Baylor athlete, is well qualified to critically analyze the dietary practices and theories that are alleged to improve performance, and has presented sound nutritional advice and recommendations for athletes, coaches, and trainers.

Since obtaining his Ph.D. in physical education at Florida State University and completing a post-doctoral study in food

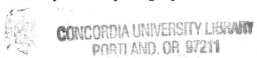

and nutrition at the same institution, Dr. Darden has been very successful in supervising training programs for athletes and executives. Many of his more than 100 published articles have been in the field of nutrition and physical development.

This book is highly recommended for all athletes, coaches, and trainers who desire to become more enlightened concerning nutrition and athletic performance.

Fred L. Allman, Jr., M.D.
Past Chairman, Committee on
Exercise and Physical Fitness
— American Medical Assn.

Sports Medicine Clinic
Atlanta, Georgia
January 5, 1976

Table of Contents

Preface

INTEREST IN nutrition has been on the upswing for the last several years. This began with the recognition that a form of malnutrition (overeating, especially of animal fats) was the main cause of heart disease. More recently, ecological issues have focused attention on the possible dangers of food contaminants and additives. Furthermore, great progress has been made during the last 50 years in the understanding of nutrition and its relationship to health and performance. This progress has provided large amounts of publicity and has also helped to make people curious about nutrition.

People, therefore, have begun to seek ways to improve their diets. With this greater interest (or demand), "health food" stores have sprung up like weeds, and movie stars and famous athletes have begun to promote all kinds of dietary supplements. Like many Americans, young athletes have also been influenced by and have become susceptible to the manufacturer of dietary supplements who is willing to use half truths and outright lies to sell his products. Questions are being continually asked by athletes and coaches concerning the effects of various dietary regimens on physical performance. Which vitamins should be taken to develop stamina? Should beef steak be eaten to promote muscle growth? What diets are best for developing strength?

The search for the magic food to increase performance is not a modern phenomenon. Early soldiers from Macedonia are said to have eaten mushrooms for this purpose. A group of Nordic soldiers are reported to have eaten a constituent of fungus to increase their endurance. Athletes in the ancient Olympic Games at the end of the third century B.C. thought they obtained great strength from eating raw meat. Similarly, athletes in the current Olympic contests eat many special diet supplements in order to gain a "hope for" advantage over their competitors.

Yes, the quest for the best diet still goes on. Cases are described of some athletes who consume green vitamin pills in the morning, yellow pills at noon, and pink ones at night. And just to be sure, they take special desiccated liver supplements "for the muscle" as well as for "quick energy." In between they munch on flavored protein pills and wash it all down with wheat germ oil.

On the one hand, it is very encouraging to see the new wave of interest in nutrition, since the diet of many Americans is atrocious and needs improvement. On the other hand, it is discouraging to see how many people will try to exploit this interest for their own personal gain, and how gullible people are to the lies and half truths exposed in "health food " stores and on television.

The question is where will it all end or what is the best course of action? We do need to learn about nutrition and select the proper diet if we are to enjoy long life and vigorous health. Objective answers to such questions are not easy to find as they must be tailor-made for each individual according to his particular situation. Moreover, many of these answers are located in scientific journals which are written in a complex fashion using words that are unfamiliar to most people.

Thus, the purpose of this book is threefold:

1. To provide a background in nutritional principles that relate to athletic performance.
2. To critically analyze some of the dietary practices and theories that are alleged to improve athletic performance.
3. To present sound nutritional advice and recommendations for all athletes, coaches, and trainers.

In this book I have referred to some of the major research studies that are relevant to nutrition and athletic performance. This research is presented in a non-technical manner. In fact, over half the book is arranged in a question and answer format. The book was written mainly for athletes, coaches, trainers, and physical educators. In most instances, however, the concepts that are presented apply to the general population. Special attention is also given to the female athlete.

Introductory material, definitions, principles of nutrition, and other background information relating to food and nutrition are considered in Chapter 1. Chapters 2 and 3 concern the determination of your nutritional status and caloric requirements. The next four chapters discuss the various classes of nutrients with special attention given to their relationship to athletic performance. Current dietary theories and practices also are referred to in this section. The various facts and fallacies of "health foods," dietary supplements, and drugs make Chapters 8 and 9 important for the coach and athlete. What about the female athlete? Don't despair. Chapter 10 is written especially for women. Finally, the last chapter presents dietary guidelines for athletic training and points out that adequate nutrition and physical activity are only two of the numerous factors that help a person achieve total health or reach his potential.

Ellington Darden

Lake Helen, Florida
March 1, 1976

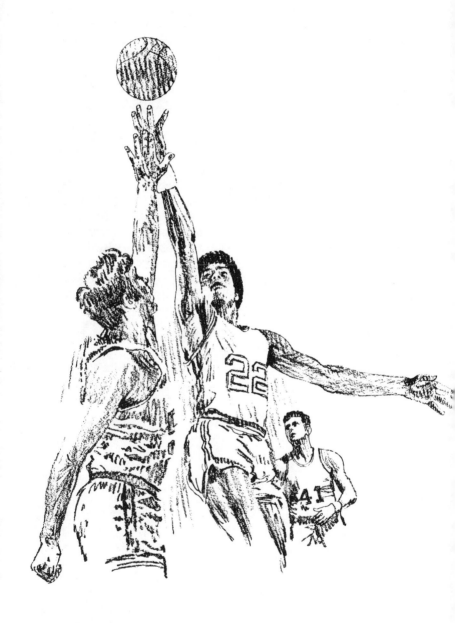

1

The Ins and Outs
of Nutrition

ALMOST EVERYONE seems to be interested in food and nutrition these days. And everyone thinks he or she is an expert; after all, haven't they been eating two to four meals a day all their lives?

With the tremendous growth in population and decrease in the number of families who grow and preserve their own food, the food-marketing industry, from the grower to the retailer, has continued to expand until it has become a multi-billion dollar operation.

More recently our scientific understanding and the publicity given to the relationship between nutrition and health has generated a whole new interest in special diets, foods, and supplements. People have been led to believe that any or all of their symptoms and ill health are due to incomplete diets or contaminated foods.

Because so much interest in nutrition has been generated and since so many people have begun to ask what they should eat, the field of nutrition has begun to offer lucrative gains for those who are willing to exploit half-truths, misinformation, and downright lies. It appears that there is a rapidly growing segment of our population whose primary interest is to sell special foods and dietary supplements and to exploit a need by whatever means seems workable, with little regard for honesty or truth.

We treat the lies expounded on TV commercials flippantly and with ridicule, but they apparently do influence many people because they have been proven to be effective. They do sell products! Such promotion and advertising leaves the consumer in an awkward and even dangerous position. The consumer has limited knowledge of the science of nutrition, but at the same time is familiar with the names of some of the nutrients that appear on the labels of the highly advertised items. Therefore the ad man readily takes advantage of the consumer's limited knowledge, distorts the facts or applies them incorrectly, and promotes his product. The well known generalization, "If a little is good, more is better" does not apply to nutrition; but, the concept "A little knowledge is a dangerous thing" surely does apply.

Within recent years, numerous coaches and athletes have become victims of many food fallacies and much nutritional misinformation. Most American athletes are willing and can afford to try almost anything to improve their performance.

Why are coaches and athletes so susceptible to this misinformation? With their drive and motivation to compete and win, they are naturally interested in any product that is supposed to improve their performance. Once an athlete begins to approach the maximum achievement possible for a particular event, he begins to search for something else to add to his training program that will give him the necessary edge over his competition.

Furthermore, athletes and coaches frequently read articles in sports magazines that describe the training program and dietary practice of champions. Sometimes the details of the training program are not accurate and at other times, the alleged benefit or the champion's success was actually not due to the special diet or dietary supplement but to various other factors. While this practice seems educational or at least harmless, it can be dangerous and damaging.

Although most of these magazines have a scientific or authentic looking format, they are in reality merely promotion magazines for various products. They contain biased reports or carefully selected statements made by well-known athletes. In addition, famous athletes are often paid for allowing their names to be used to promote the sale of certain products. It is unfortunate that famous athletes and TV advertisements have so much influence on Americans' eating habits. Obviously, the place to go for information about nutrition is not a paid athlete's statements or a TV commercial designed to sell a particular product.

The coach and athlete must be aware of at least some of the fallacies that are prevalent concerning food and nutrition. Food fallacies can be considered in several categories. One type of fallacy arises merely as a custom, without specific regard to nutritional value.

A second category is that which attaches special virtues to a particular food or diet. Another category of the special virtue type is the distortion of the relative importance of proteins, vitamins, and minerals. A fourth group of fallacies emphasizes "natural" or "health foods" as opposed to processed foods. To these four groups, a fifth and final category that has recently become a problem, is the use and effects of various "drugs" for improving performance. Each of these five catagories will be discussed in detail in the succeeding chapters.

While many of the alleged benefits of special diets and dietary supplements are not accurately stated, correct nutrition for the athlete can mean the difference between having enough stamina and tiring halfway through a game; or between a sense of well-being and a feeling or not being up to par. It can also make the difference between winning and losing. Of course, factors other than diet can affect performance, but taking nutrition for granted or the indiscriminant use of dietary supplements, may produce an unnecessary handicap or be dangerous to health.

What is the best way to attack the problems of food and nutritional misinformation and fallacies? Education and understanding, whereby accurate authoritative information is supplied, should be the principle weapons. Nutrition facts must be kept before the public. Although the answers to some questions regarding optimum nutrition are unknown, the health of a great majority of Americans would be vastly improved if our current knowledge of nutrition was accurately applied.

WHAT IS NUTRITION?

Nutrition is a science. That is, it is made up of a body of systematized knowledge or facts, which have been established according to the scientific or experimental method. The scientific disciplines can be divided into the natural and the social sciences. Nutrition belongs to the group of natural sciences or those that concern nature and the physical world. Natural sciences may be divided into those described as pure: such as mathematics, physics, chemistry and biology; and those described as applied: such as engineering, medicine, nutrition, agriculture, and geology.

To some people, nutrition refers to the preparation and service of tasty foods in an attractive manner. Although nutrition begins with food, it surely doesn't end there. To others, nutrition refers more to various agricultural practices used in the growth and development of healthy, marketable livestock. To others, it refers to cell processes and how cells receive their required nutrients. Actually it includes all of these.

Nutrition is both a scientific discipline and a biological process. For the purpose of this book, which is concerned almost totally with human nutrition, the word *nutrition* is defined as *the study of the food we eat and how the body uses it*. Nutrition is a process in which food is ingested and digested, its nutrients absorbed and distributed to cells in all parts of the body. Here they are either used, and extra amounts stored, or they are excreted along with the unabsorbed food debris and the waste products of the body processes. Therefore, the attainment of nutritional status is dependent on the performance of many integrated systems in the body.

This nutritional process may be successful, or it may be faulty in varying degrees at different points. Faulty nutrition or malnutrition may result from the consumption of too little or too much food, the wrong kinds of food, or from a functional failure in one or more systems of the body. Such a functional failure in one or more steps through which food passes before it is ready for cell use and finally excretion, may render the diet partially or completely ineffective.

Various terms have been used by laymen to describe the quality of a subject's nutritional state, such as: poor nutrition, faulty nutrition, inadequate nutrition, etc. Actually, there are three general categories which are used by nutritionalists to describe the nutritional status of a subject: undernutrition, optimum nutrition, and overnutrition. The first and the last of these states can be described as types of malnutrition (poor nutrition). Obviously, undernutrition of one or all nutrients may also lead to ill health and disease, or obesity with all of its complications. Today far more Americans suffer from ill health due to overnutrition than from deficiency states of undernutrition; in fact, more Americans die from a disease of overnutrition (heart disease) than all other diseases combined.

Although food is the basic factor in preventing malnutrition, one must learn how to select the right foods, prepare them correctly, and consume them in the proper amount and at the right time in order to achieve optimum nutrition.

NUTRIENT CLASSIFICATION

Food is composed of various chemical compounds called nutrients. Nutrients are necessary for the proper functioning of the body and therefore must be provided to every cell and tissue. There are at least fifty nutrients that can be classified in the following groups according to their similarity of chemical structure or function:

1. Carbohydrates
2. Fats or lipids
3. Proteins
4. Vitamins
5. Minerals
6. Water

By far, the most abundant nutrients in foods are carbohydrates, fats, proteins, and water. Almost all of the total weight of foods is composed of these four nutrients. Vitamins and minerals occur in much smaller quantities and yet they are equally important for the proper operation of all cells. The six classes of nutrients serve the body in three general ways: (1) to provide energy for activities and heat to maintain body temperatures, (2) for growth and maintenance, and (3) to control and coordinate the internal processes. All nutrients serve the body in one or more of these capacities or functions.

Few foods are all carbohydrates or all protein or all fat. The common ones are table syrups and sugar (all carbohydrate); cooking oils (all fat); and plain, unflavored gelatin (nearly all protein). Almost all other foods you eat are made up of a mixture of all the nutrients.

ESSENTIAL AND NON-ESSENTIAL NUTRIENTS

The nutrients can be further separated into essential and non-essential groups. An essential nutrient is one that cannot be synthesized from simpler materials (ordinarily present in the diet) at a sufficient rate for optimum health and therefore must be supplied in the diet. Non-essential nutrients are also needed by the cells, but can be synthesized in the body from simpler materials (provided in the diet or from the breakdown of other cell components). However, for the most efficient operation of cell metabolism and body function both essential and non-essential nutrients should be present in the diet.

Essential Nutrients (must be present in the diet)

1. Sources of energy: carbohydrates or fats
2. Polyunsaturated fatty acid or linoleic acid
3. Threonine
4. Tryptophan
5. Lysine
6. Leucine
7. Iso-leucine
8. Methionine
9. Valine
10. Phenylalamine
11. Histidine (may be essential for infants)
12. Arginine (may be essential for adults)
13. Vitamin A
14. Vitamin D
15. Vitamin E
16. Vitamin K
17. Ascorbic Acid (Vitamin C)
18. Thiamin
19. Riboflavin
20. Niacin
21. Pyridoxine
22. Folic Acid
23. Pantothenic Acid
24. Biotin
25. Vitamin B_{12}
26. Calcium
27. Phosphorus
28. Sodium
29. Chloride
30. Potassium
31. Magnesium
32. Iron
33. Copper
34. Manganese

35. Iodine
36. Cobalt
37. Zinc
38. Fluoride
39. Molybdenum
40. Selenium
41. Chromium
42. Water

Some of the Non-Essential Nutrients (required by the cells)

43. Carbohydrates
44. Fats
45. Choline
46. Glycine
47. Alanine
48. Cysteine
49. Cystine
50. Serine
51. Tyrosine
52. Aspartic Acid
53. Glutamic Acid
54. Proline
55. Hydroxyproline

There are many other compounds that are required by the body for its normal function or operation. These compounds can be made by the cells from the by-products or end products of metabolism or from other nutrients present in the diet. Although the non-essential nutrients can be made in the body, it would prefer to ingest them. Such a diet would require less work or effort by the cells and therefore would provide for the most efficient operation of the cells.

PROCESSES CONCERNED WITH FOOD UTILIZATION

When a steak or vegetable salad is eaten, the nutrients from these foods will eventually be used to feed or nourish the cells of your body. Before the nutrients contained in these foods can actually reach the cells, the foods must be digested and the nutrients absorbed. During digestion, food is reduced to very simple forms or smaller molecules that can be dissolved or suspended in liquids. These liquids with the suspended nutrients can then enter the body through the tiny holes or pores in the intestinal wall. After absorption, the nutrients travel in the blood and lymph to all cells of the body. As the nutrients pass by the cells, the cells drink in those particular nutrients they happen to need at that moment, for use in carrying out their functions (by entering into the chemical reactions of the cell).

DIGESTION

The digestive tract is composed of the mouth, esophagus, stomach, small intestine, and large intestine (see Figure 1.1). The mechanical and chemical phases of digestion occur in these organs. The mechanical phase of digestion, which is responsible for the subdividing, mixing, and propelling of the food mass along the digestive tract, is brought about by chewing in the mouth, the act of swallowing, and muscular activity of the walls of the tract itself. The chemical phase of digestion, which is responsible for the final breakdown of food particles, is brought about by the action of a group of substances called digestive enzymes. Enzymes act as catalysts in the body; that is, they increase the rate of a reaction without becoming part of the final reaction product. In this case, the enzymes aid in the breakdown of the complex of large nutrient molecules to smaller molecules. For example, carbohydrates are changed into simple sugars, the fats to glycerol and fatty acids, and the proteins to amino acids.

The process of digestion starts when food enters your body through the mouth where it is chewed, broken into small pieces, and mixed with saliva. The fluid secreted by the salivary glands contains some digestive enzymes which act on carbohydrates. From the mouth, the food then passes to the stomach by way of the esophagus. The digestion of certain food continues in the stomach under the influence of the secretions and churning action of the stomach wall. Ordinarily a mixed meal leaves the stomach in three to four and one-half hours; however, this time can vary according to the composition of the diet. Carbohydrates leave the stomach most rapidly, followed by proteins, while fats remain in the stomach for the longest length of time. Thus, the sensation of hunger occurs sooner after a meal relatively high in carbohydrate than after a meal containing adequate amounts of protein or fat.

After leaving the stomach, the liquified food mass, called chyme, passes into the small intestine which is a coiled tube

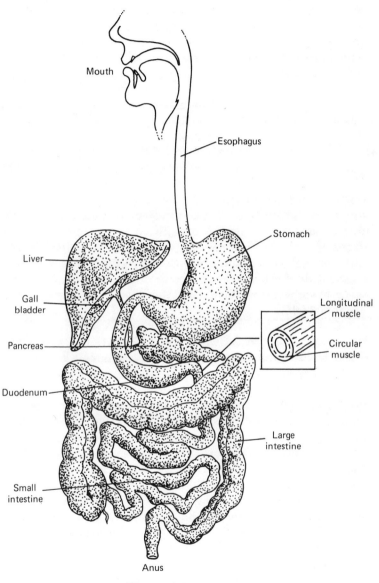

Figure 1.1
THE DIGESTIVE TRACT.

over 20 feet in length. The final digestion of food particles occurs in the small intestine under the influence of secretions from its walls and from the liver and pancreas which pour their secretions into the small intestine through little tubes or ducts. The undigested food residues pass from the small intestine into the large intestine or colon. This material also contains some of the end products of digestion such as water, as well as waste materials. These waste products pass through the large intestine and are stored in the rectum where they await periodic excretion from the body.

ABSORPTION

Absorption is closely related to digestion since the function of digestion is to prepare the nutrients for absorption through the walls of the digestive tract. Most of this absorption takes place in the small intestine, although water and small amounts of simple sugars and alcohol pass through the mucosa of the stomach into the blood stream, while various minerals and water are absorbed in the large intestine. Fingerlike projections on the wall of the intestines into the "food canal," called *villi,* favor absorption by increasing the absorptive surface area about 600 fold.

CIRCULATION AND RESPIRATION

Each villus contains a network of tiny vessels which drink up the nutrients as they pass along the food canal. Actually there are two kinds of tiny vessels in each villus: one that contains lymph and accepts digested fats (lymphatic vessels) and the other that contains blood and accepts all other digested nutrients (capillaries). Since these litle vessels are part of the body's circulatory system, they are the means or route by which the absorbed nutrients are circulated to every cell in every tissue and organ throughout the body.

The lungs represent another route of entry for the very important cell nutrient: oxygen. Analogous to the villi in the intestines, are the *alveoli* in the lungs. These alveoli are tiny projections into the "air canal" and like the intestinal villi, they contain a network of tiny vessels (capillaries) which contain blood and which drink up the oxygen as it is inhaled into the lungs.

The nutrient molecules and the oxygen are then circulated throughout the body and are accepted by the cells according to their need as the blood flows by, much like a mechanical cafeteria. Those nutrients and that amount of oxygen which are not needed by the cells for immediate use, are available to various other cells for storage. Since most cells have a limit on how much of a particular nutrient or oxygen they can hold, the remainder is converted into other materials or compounds that can be stored or is excreted from the body.

Since food as consumed is of no use to the body, it must first be broken down into smaller pieces so it can be swallowed, and then digested into smaller molecules so it can be absorbed to feed the cells.

For example, a carrot contains several vitamins; especially a form of vitamin A, some starch that is a form of carbohydrate, some poor-quality protein, several minerals, and water. Once the carrot has been digested and its nutrients are absorbed and transported to the cells, they are accepted according to need and function of that particular cell. The vitamin A would be accepted for use in the retina of the eye, by various other cells throughout the body, or picked up by the liver for storage. The starch digested to glucose would be picked up by any cell in the body to be used as an energy source, or stored in the liver or muscle as glycogen (storage form of carbohydrate), or if the glycogen stores were filled it would be picked up by the fat storage cells where it is converted to and stored as fat. The protein digested to amino acids would be used or converted to glycogen or fat for storage. The minerals would be picked up for use and the extra amounts would either be accepted by cells or excreted by the kidneys in the urine.

METABOLISM

Once the cell accepts a nutrient, it is carried to certain parts of the cell where it enters into various chemical reactions. In general, these reactions are either constructive (anabolic), or degradative (catabolic). The constructive reactions would be associated with growth, pregnancy, lactation, healing, etc. The degradative reactions would be associated with the release of energy when nutrients are "burned" or broken down during infections, or muscle wasting, and during the continuous destruction of worn-out cells. Of course both processes go on simultaneously in different parts or cells of the body.

Each cell in the body can be considered a microscopic part of the whole organism. It must receive a source of energy (typically carbohydrates and fats), oxygen (for use in releasing the energy from the carbohydrates and fats), vitamins, amino acids and minerals for use in making enzymes (the catalysts for its reactions), and the other necessary cell components that are needed to maintain the cell and carry out the functions assigned to it. Each cell must be protected and kept warm, it must be able to rid itself of its waste products, it must be sensitive and able to react to various stimuli. It is born, matures, lives for a while, dies, and is broken down with certain parts, reused and the rest carried off for excretion.

In short, the human body is the most complex machine on earth. Man has never been able to create a machine that is comparable to his body, or to completely understand the complex interaction of all these components in building, maintaining, and regulating the body processes.

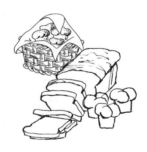

2

Your Nutritional Status How Do You Rate?

To MAKE A thorough assessment of your nutritional status it is necessary to view the task as a series of evaluations applied to the body as a whole or to body areas sensitive to nutritional measurements. Reduced to the simplest terms, such evaluations are a measure of an individual's body structure and how he looks, feels, and functions. For example, a person in excellent nutritional status from birth can be expected: (1) to have a well-developed skeleton, with well-formed teeth and jaws, (2) to exhibit a normal padding of fat over bones and muscles, and (3) to have a blood supply that carries adequate amounts of oxygen and nutrients to the cells. It is safe to predict that most people with these basic characteristics of good nutritional status will also be likely to display outward signs of vigor and health.

Determining your nutritional status requires sophisticated measuring techniques. Of course, these techniques are designed for use by specialists in various scientific fields. However, several of these methods and present standards for their use will be briefly described. Hopefully you will be able to grasp how each type of evaluation contributes to a comprehensive assessment of your nutritional status.

PHYSICIAL EXAMINATION

The first step in the assessment of your nutritional status is a general physical examination. Physicians are aware that many nutritional deficiencies may be (but are not always) expressed by some of the following superficial signs and symptoms: stiff and brittle hair; abnormally dry and rough skin; dry, dull, lusterless eyes, with irritated lids; a deep red and fissured tongue; spongy and bleeding gums; and lips that are swollen, chapped, and cracked at the corners.

The second step in the assessment of nutritional status should be the measurement of the body to perform its various functions. For example: color vision, vision in dim light, heart function, and work capacity.

Since these gross clinical signs and functions are easy to observe, they are often used in making the initial tentative estimate of an individual's nutritional status. However, they are general signs of ill health and therefore do not necessarily indicate malnutrition. Malnutrition can also be provoked by non-dietary factors such as infection or by faulty digestion, absorption, utilization or elimination.

The following diagram by the well-known British nutritionist, Dr. H. M. Sinclair, points out that your physical well-being is composed of many interrelated factors:

This diagram indicates the complex nature of body condition and the difficulty in assessing it.

HEIGHT AND WEIGHT

Desirable height and weight charts have been devised for men and women. These averages are found in Table 2-1. Although it is difficult to state ideal weights, these tables present typical ranges of body weight among apparently healthy individuals according to height, age, sex, and frame (size and weight of skeleton). However, the drawbacks to these charts are that they don't apply to many athletes, especially those who are very muscular. For example, a fullback on a football team may be six-feet tall and weigh 200 pounds with little excess fat. But according to the chart he would be from 17 to 46 pounds over-

26

weight. Obviously the charts do not account for muscle hypertrophy. Rather they are averages of the general population. Since overweight or more specifically "over fat" is known to be unhealthy or undesirable, a better method of determining the body fat of an athlete would be to use specific measurement of body fat.

TABLE 2-1
WEIGHTS FOR HEIGHTS OF MEN AND WOMEN

Height	Weights for Men			Weights for Women		
	Low	Median	High	Low	Median	High
Inches	Pounds	Pounds	Pounds	Pounds	Pounds	Pounds
60	------	------	------	100	109	118
61	------	------	------	104	112	121
62	------	------	------	107	115	125
63	118	129	141	110	118	128
64	122	133	145	113	122	132
65	126	137	149	116	125	135
66	130	142	155	120	129	139
67	134	147	161	123	132	142
68	139	151	166	126	136	146
69	143	155	170	130	140	151
70	147	159	174	133	144	156
71	150	163	178	137	148	161
72	154	167	183	141	152	166
73	158	171	188	------	------	------
74	162	175	192	------	------	------
75	165	178	195	------	------	------

BODY FAT

A person is said to be obese (excessively overweight) when his body weight is 20 percent greater than his ideal weight. Several methods have been used to measure body fat, namely: x-rays, specific gravity, "potassium 40", and skin-fold thickness. The easiest and most popular method of assessing the amount of body fat is by measuring skin-fold thickness. The thickness of a fold of skin in various areas of the body (e.g., triceps, abdomen, hips, thighs, etc.) is measured with skin-fold calipers. Such thickness data can be translated into percentage of body fat. Although these data are not perfect or totally precise, they do give a better indication of amount of body fat than mere body weight and height data. Typically the amount of body fat varies with age and sex. In general, it is greatest in infancy and diminishes in childhood and increases again during adolescence. Research indicates that girls and women normally have more body fat than do boys and men. An abnormally great or small amount of body fat is related to poor nutritional status. Standards to aid in determining when the amount of body fat is abnormal are presented in Table 2-2. The table also indicates that the amount of fat in the tricep area varies throughout life.

TABLE 2-2
OBESITY STANDARDS FOR CAUCASIAN AMERICANS
Minimum triceps skinfold thickness in millimeters

Age (years)	Skinfold measurements	
	Males	Females
5	12	14
6	12	15
7	13	16
8	14	17
9	15	18
10	16	20
11	17	21
12	18	22
13	18	23
14	17	23
15	16	24
16	15	25
17	14	26
18	15	27
19	15	27
20	16	28
21	17	28
22	18	28
23	18	28
24	19	28
25	20	29
26	20	29
27	21	29
28	22	29
29	23	29
30—50	23	30

Most Americans have over 20 percent of their body weight in the form of fat. And as you would expect, athletes have a smaller percentage of fat than non-athletes. Table 2-3 shows the results of a study recently completed on Czechoslovakian athletes. You will notice that most of these athletes have a minimum amount of body fat. In fact, seldom do you find successful male athletes with more than 12 percent body fat.

TABLE 2-3
BODY WEIGHT AND FATNESS OF 10 MEN AND 10 WOMEN CHAMPIONS IN DIFFERENT SPORTS

MEN	Weight (lbs.)	% Body Fat
1. Gymnastics	148.7	4.5
2. Marathon runners	135.7	6.1
3. Weight lifting	170.3	6.2
4. Racing cycling	155.8	6.2
5. Tennis	138.2	7.3
6. Volleyball	174.7	7.5
7. Table tennis	128.7	9.2
8. Basketball	215.8	11.7
9. Ice hockey	148.1	14.8
10. Greco-Roman wrestling	227.0	19.0
WOMEN		
1. Gymnastics	122.3	8.3
2. Gymnastics	117.7	10.2
3. High jump	136.8	10.3
4. 10 m diving	110.0	12.4
5. Skiing 10 km	120.1	13.5
6. Swimming	153.6	13.8
7. Ice skating	128.3	15.3
8. Tennis	137.5	18.2
9. Table tennis	115.3	18.3
10. Shot put and discus	179.7	19.7

COMPOSITION OF BLOOD AND URINE

A more precise but expensive way of assessing a person's nutritional status is to measure the nutrients circulating in the blood or being excreted in the urine. Such measurements actually reveal the tissue status of the nutrients and can be judged to be normal by comparison with data from healthy, well-nourished individuals of the same sex, age, physical development, and activity.

FOOD HABITS AND DIET RECORDS

How does the athlete know if he is eating correctly? Until he keeps a daily record of his eating habits, he probably doesn't realize how much of particular foods he consumes. In this respect, you are urged to "keep score" on the details of your diet. You need to record how much of each food you consume for several days — both on weekdays and on weekends. This will tell you which of your eating habits need improvement; the frequency of eating as well as the quality (nutrient content) and

TABLE 2-4
COMPARATIVE DIETARY STANDARDS OF SELECTED COUNTRIES AND U.N. AGENCIES

Country	Sex	Age (years)	Weight (kg)	kcal	Protein (g)	Calcium (mg)	Iron (mg)	Vit. A activity (IU)	Thiamin (mg)	Riboflavin (mg)	Niacin equiv. (mg)	Ascorbic acid (mg)
U.S.A.	M	22	70	2,800	52	800	10	5,000	1.5	1.8	20	45
	F	22	58	2,000	46	800	18	4,000	1.1	1.4	14	45
FAO-WHO	M	25	65	3,200	46	400-500			1.3	1.8	21.1	
	F	25	65	2,300	39	400-500			0.9	1.3	15.2	
Australia	M	25	70	2,900	70	400-800	10	2,500	1.2	1.5	18	30
	F	25	58	2,100	58	400-800	10	2,500	0.8	1.1	14	30
Colombia	M	20-29	65	2,850	68	500	10	5,000	1.1	1.7	13.8	50
	F	20-29	55	1,900	60	500	15	5,000	0.8	1.1	12.5	50
Japan	M	26-29	56	3,000	70	600	10	2,000	1.5	1.5	15	65
	F	26-29	49	2,400	60	600	10	2,000	1.2	1.2	12	60
Norway	M	25	70	3,400	70	800	12	2,500	1.7	1.8	17	30
	F	25	60	2,500	60	800	12	2,500	1.3	1.5	13	30
Philippines	M	none specified	53	2,400	53	500		5,000	1.2	1.2		70
	F		46	1,800	46	500		5,000	0.9	0.9		70
West Germany	M	25	72	2,500	72	800	10	5,000	1.7	1.8	18	75
	F	25	60	2,200	60	800	12	5,000	1.5	1.8	14	75

quantity of the food consumed.

A thorough discussion of how to evaluate your dietary habits as well as how to select appropriate foods for your particular need is presented in Chapter 3.

RECOMMENDED DIETARY STANDARDS

The nutrients required by man are widely distributed in common foods so that many very different diets provide adequate amounts of all the nutrients. For various reasons however, some people restrict the number of different foods eaten: finicky eaters, "health food" and other food faddists consume large amounts of certain foods, and poor people consume high-carbohydrate foods because they are the least expensive. In order to help people eat the required nutrients in sufficient amounts, dietary standards have been established in many countries. These standards have been developed with the requirements of the people of each particular country in mind; the effects which cooking has on the nutritional value of the food; the digestibility and rate of absorption; and the expected variation in nutrient quality of the food. In Table 2-4, there is listed several suggested dietary allowances established for young men and women by several countries. Recommendations have also been made for people in other age groups. You will note that all of these recommendations are similar to those established for Americans by the National Research Council (see Table 2-5).

QUESTIONS AND ANSWERS CONCERNING NUTRITIONAL STATUS

Question: **What is meant when the label of a food product says that one serving or 100 grams of the food supplies a certain proportion of the M.D.R. of a particular nutrient?**

Answer: The Federal Food and Drug Administration has the responsibility of approving the labels of all foods and of food supplements for special dietary uses. Before 1974 the FDA required that nutrient contents be expressed in terms of the Minimum Daily Requirements (M.D.R.). In this respect, the contents were stated per serving, per 100 grams, or per recommended dosage.

One M.D.R. is the minimum or actual amount of the nutrient required by the body under ideal conditions. Thus, if a serving of

FOOD AND NUTRITION BOARD, NATIONAL A
COUNCIL RECOMMENDED DAILY D
Designed for the Maintenance of Good Nutriti

FAT-SOLUBLE VITAMIN

	(years) From/Up to	Weight (lbs)	Height (in)	Energy (kcal)	Protein (g)	Vit. A activity (IU)	Vit. D (IU)	Vit. E activity (IU)
INFANTS	0.0-0.5	14	24	x 117	kg x 2.2	1,400	400	4
	0.5-1.0	20	28	x 108	kg x 2.0	2,000	400	5
CHILDREN	1-3	28	34	1300	23	2,000	400	7
	4-6	44	44	1800	30	2,500	400	9
	7-10	66	54	2400	36	3,300	400	10
MALES	11-14	97	63	2800	44	5,000	400	12
	15-18	134	69	3000	54	5,000	400	15
	19-22	147	69	3000	52	5,000	400	15
	23-50	154	69	2700	56	5,000	--	15
	51 +	154	69	2400	56	5,000	--	15
FEMALES	11-14	97	62	2400	44	4,000	400	10
	15-18	119	65	2100	48	4,000	400	11
	19-22	128	65	2100	46	4,000	400	12
	23-50	128	65	2000	46	4,000	--	12
	51 +	128	65	1800	46	4,000	--	12
PREGNANCY	--	--	--	+300	+30	5,000	400	15
LACTATION	--	--	--	+500	+20	6,000	400	15

A. The allowances are intended to provide for individual variations among most normal pe
on a variety of common foods in order to provide other nutrients for which human req
2. Microgram.
3. This increased requirement cannot be met by ordinary diets; therefore, the use of supp

food provides half of the body's actual or minimum requirement of vitamin A for the healthy subject living under the best conditions, the label would indicate that one serving supplies 50 percent of the M.D.R. for vitamin A. The manufacturer's label may also list the contents of nutrients not required by man. In these cases, the label must state that a M.D.R. for that particular nutrient has not been established for man.

Recently, however, the FDA put into effect revised nutrient label requirements that center around the Recommended Dietary Allowances rather than the Minimum Daily Requirements.

Question: **What does the term "Recommended Dietary Allowances" mean? Is it a good standard for determining the amount of nutrients required by athletes?**

Answer: The Recommended Dietary Allowances (R.D.A.) were first established by the Food and Nutrition Board of the

ATER-SOLUBLE VITAMINS   MINERALS

or- ic id g)	Fola- cin (μg)²	Nia- cin (mg)	Ribo- flavin (mg)	Thia- min (mg)	Vit. B6 (mg)	Vit. B12 (μg)	Cal- cium (mg)	Phos- phorus (mg)	Io- dine (μg)	Iron (mg)	Mag- ne- sium (mg)	Zinc (mg)
5	50	5	0.4	0.3	0.3	0.3	360	240	35	10	60	3
5	50	8	0.6	0.5	0.4	0.3	540	400	45	15	70	5
0	100	9	0.8	0.7	0.6	1.0	800	800	60	15	150	10
0	200	12	1.1	0.9	0.9	1.5	800	800	80	10	200	10
0	300	16	1.2	1.2	1.2	2.0	800	800	110	10	250	10
5	400	18	1.5	1.4	1.6	3.0	1200	1200	130	18	350	15
5	400	20	1.8	1.5	1.8	3.0	1200	1200	150	18	400	15
5	400	20	1.8	1.5	2.0	3.0	800	800	140	10	350	15
5	400	18	1.6	1.4	2.0	3.0	800	800	130	10	350	15
5	400	16	1.5	1.2	2.0	3.0	800	800	110	10	350	15
5	400	16	1.3	1.2	1.6	3.0	1200	1200	115	18	300	15
5	400	14	1.4	1.1	2.0	3.0	1200	1200	115	18	300	15
5	400	14	1.4	1.1	2.0	3.0	800	800	100	18	300	15
5	400	13	1.2	1.0	2.0	3.0	800	800	100	18	300	15
5	400	12	1.1	1.0	2.0	3.0	800	800	80	10	300	15
0	800	+2	+0.3	+0.3	2.5	4.0	1200	1200	125	18+³	450	20
0	600	+4	+0.5	+0.3	2.5	4.0	1200	1200	150	18	450	25

as they live in the United States under usual environmental stresses. Diets should be based
nts have been less well defined.

al iron is recommended.

National Research Council in 1940 and are revised every five years as new research data is collected. The R.D.A. are the amounts of particular nutrients that are recommended to be consumed each day. They are listed according to the age and sex of healthy subjects living in the United States. These recommendations provide for the maintenance of excellent nutritional status and therefore are recommended as goals for the nutrient intake of all healthy Americans. Although the R.D.A. are based on man's minimum daily requirements, they also include a very ample margin of safety to provide for variations in the nutrient content of the foods, the damaging effect of improper cooking procedures, the digestibility and percentage of absorption of the various nutrients, and different amounts of physical activity.

In the words of the Food and Nutrition Board, the R.D.A. "...are meant to afford a margin of sufficiency above minimal

33

requirements and are planned to provide a buffer against the needs of various stresses and to make possible other potential improvements of growth and function." Hence, the R.D.A. were designed to provide for maintenance of good nutrition not only for the average person, but for all healthy persons including athletes. It is conceivable that the stresses imposed by a vigorous conditioning program may exceed those provided by the R.D.A., but such a situation would be very rare and only temporary. This explains why it isn't justifiable for an athlete to consume a diet which is double or triple the R.D.A. (by using multivitamin, protein or mineral supplements.)

You must use judgement in using the R.D.A. to evaluate the adequacy of your dietary intake. Failure to meet the R.D.A. shouldn't be equated with malnutrition. Remember that the R.D.A. are not requirements but generous allowances. However, when you fall one-third below the R.D.A. of a particular nutrient over a period of several weeks or more you should find out why and make the necessary corrections in your eating habits.

The ultimate evaluation of your nutritional status requires more than casual observation. Feeling "below par" isn't sufficient evidence to justify the conclusion that you are malnourished. Inadequate rest, illness, or emotional stresses can also rob athletes of their vitality. If you achieve the goals set by the R.D.A., however, you can be assured of being well-nourished unless you have some physical abnormality or disease.

Question: **The word "balance" is used in so many ways in nutrition (e.g., balanced diet, caloric balance, vitamin and mineral balance). What does it mean?**

Answer: The term "balanced diet" is a phrase that refers to a diet providing all of the nutrients required by a person depending on his sex, age, activity and physiological condition (healthy, pregnant, etc.). Since no single food provides all of the 50 or more required nutrients in the proper amount, the balanced diet is usually made up of many different foods and therefore is often said to be a "mixed diet."

The most noteworthy efforts to simplify the achievement of a balanced diet have been the development of the Recommended Dietary Allowances and the grouping of foods. The "Basic Four" food groups are: (1) meat, fish, and poultry with nuts and legumens as alternates, (2) milk and milk products, (3) fruits and vegetables and, (4) bread and cereals. Selection of food from each group in the recommended amounts will provide a balanced or adequate diet.

When the term balance is used in phrases like caloric balance or calcium balance, it refers to intake versus output (expenditure or need). Again the goal is to supply the body's requirements by replacing the nutrients used up or lost from the body without storing any great "excess baggage." An athlete is in caloric balance when the number of calories consumed equals the number expended. On the other hand, an athlete would be in positive caloric balance when he is gaining weight due to the storage of fat.

At some times it is desirable to be in a positive balance for certain nutrients, while at other times, it is best to be in a negative balance, while at still other times it is best to be in equilibrium. For example, one must be in a negative caloric balance in order to lose fat, in a positive calcium balance during bone growth or healing, and in equilibrium for most nutrients in adulthood.

Question: **How can an athlete really tell whether he is well-nourished? Is there a simple way of determining nutritional status?**

Answer: Since good nutrition is a prerequisite to good health, then indications of poor health may indicate poor nutrition. A good look in a full-length mirror can give a very subjective and approximate overall estimate of nutritional status. If you are either too fat or too thin in appearance, you may be improperly nourished.

However, these are usually very crude estimates of nutritional status ... since they assume that all sickness is due to malnutrition and that you know what "too fat" or "too thin" looks like. Often our concept of a healthy figure is dictated by cultural fads and not optimum health. Furthermore, appearance does not always reveal muscle tone or when the amount of body fat is excessive.

Most of the time, you should have a general feeling of vitality and well-being. You should feel alert and have the energy needed to perform regular physical activities and to react to and recover quickly from stressful situations, such as disease and infection. (However, fatigue caused by lack of sufficient rest shouldn't be confused with that caused by poor nutrition). Your

35

appetite should be good and you should have a cheerful, rather than an irritable or defeated outlook on life's situations. Height and weight should be normal for your inherited body build when compared to other healthy persons of the same age and sex.

Although the feeling of well-being and one's physical appearance give a general indication of nutritional status, they do not tell for sure whether you are eating an adequate diet or in which nutrients it is deficient. More specific tests for measuring nutritional adequacy are described in the first part of this chapter.

Question: **What is the difference between the M.D.R. and the R.D.A.?**

Answer: Much confusion exists among the general population concerning the use of the terms Minimum Daily Requirements (M.D.R.) and the Recommended Dietary Allowances (R.D.A.). The Minimum Daily Requirement (M.D.R.) refers to the actual or minimum amount of a nutrient required by the body each day *when all other conditions are ideal*. The Recommended Dietary Allowances (R.D.A.) are based on these minimum requirements, but then recommend that an extra amount of the nutrient should be present in the diet in order to be sure the person receives adequate nourishment *when all other conditions are not ideal*. For example, if you eat a diet that just meets the M.D.R. for all nutrients, it would not be adequate to account for any of the loss of nutrients due to cooking, suboptimum digestion and absorption (brought about by many causes), or if your requirements are increased during minor infections or illness, growth, pregnancy, lactation, or rehabilitation from disease. On the other hand, the R.D.A. is more generous, safe, and satisfactory guide for use in formulating adequate diets.

Naturally the food industry prefers to use the smaller M.D.R. in their advertising programs. (And this specifically is why the FDA is promoting the use of RDA's in their new labeling programs.) For example a certain cereal company says that two ounces of their cereal contains 100 percent of the M.D.R. of vitamin C. In other words, the minimum requirement for vitamin C is 10 milligrams per day and two ounces of the advertised cereal would provide 10 mg. On the other hand, the recommended intake of vitamin C for adults is 45 mg. which would be provided in ten ounces of the above cereal. Don't be misled by thinking that M.D.R. and R.D.A. stand for the same thing or are equivalent.

Question: **Do all athletes have the same nutrient requirements?**

Answer: Athletes don't have identical nutrient requirements. In fact, the amount of nutrients you require can change from day to day. But this change is quite small. The greatest difference in nutrient requirements between athletes is the difference in energy expenditure required by the particular athletic event. Men and women who participate in endurance events, such as distance running, have different requirements than those engaged in strength events, such as weightlifters. The nutrient requirements for a six-foot four-inch, 165 pound golfer are quite different from those of a six-foot four-inch, 240 pound defensive tackle. The R.D.A. represent an excellent starting point for determining what your nutrient intake should be, but you will have to determine whether they suit your particular event and body build.

Information is available that permits reasonably accurate estimates of an athlete's nutrient requirements based on age, sex, body size, and physical activity. Other factors that must be considered in determining specific nutrient requirements are: growth, pregnancy, illness, environmental temperature, efficiency of food digestion, and nutrient absorption.

Question: **Why is breakfast such an important meal for the athlete?**

Answer: Breakfast is considered an important meal because it marks the end of an overnight fast. Studies made on the value of breakfast have shown that performance during the late morning hours is impaired in those individuals who skip breakfast.

In many cases, the coffee break or midmorning snack has been substituted for breakfast. A study was made to determine if any discernable difference could be shown between the performance of workers who ate breakfast and those who ate only a midmorning snack. Here again, it was observed that a snack in the middle of the morning didn't adequately replace a good breakfast in approximately half of the subjects who participated in the study. The individuals who ate a good breakfast did much more work in the late morning hours than those who omitted breakfast. Such differences were apparent even in the subjects who were relatively sedentary and whose activities and requirements were small.

Therefore, breakfast would be very important for the athlete who is engaged in rigorous physical activity and who must maintain a high level of nutrition if he is to compete at his maximum capability. He will never achieve these goals if he must recover from a nutritional slump that he puts himself into each morning.

The size of the breakfast depends on the athlete's total nutrient requirements. It has been recommended that breakfast should supply at least 25 percent of your nutrient needs for the day. So practice eating breakfast — it'll pay off!

Question: **Are the new liquid or instant breakfasts nourishing?**

Answer: Liquid or instant breakfasts supply reasonable quantities of most of the nutrients needed by man. These breakfasts are available in a powder to be mixed with milk or as a can of ready-mixed product.

One can or the contents of an envelope mixed with eight fluid ounces of whole milk will provide about 300 calories and 17 to 18 grams of protein. While the vitamin and mineral contents vary somewhat among products, they are designed to provide from 25 to 33 percent of the day's needs for nutrients, except calories. Nevertheless, when the choice exists between an instant breakfast and a balanced breakfast of milk, cereal, fruit, and meat, the latter is superior in many respects: flavor, bulk, and satisfaction.

Question: **What proportion of the daily caloric need should be consumed with each meal?**

Answer: There is little agreement on the proportion of calories that should be consumed at the three conventional meals. The usual pattern for most people in the United States is a light breakfast and moderate lunch, followed by a heavy evening meal. Custom, work schedule, and personal preference seem to dictate meal patterns.

Actually there is a wide range in eating habits, including the spacing of meals, which occurs throughout America and around the world. In primitive and poorer societies, fewer meals are consumed, with the typical pattern often being one evening meal and chance snacks throughout the day. Although these people seem to survive and reproduce themselves, their infant mortality rate is very high, their general health is very poor, and their life span is short.

On the other hand, people in affluent societies are generally over-fed and under-active. For somewhat different reasons, their health and life span are also very suboptimal. A common habit that many overweight and under-active people have, is that of snacking throughout the day, having a couple of drinks before dinner and then eating large quantities of very rich and fatty food at the evening meal. Such a pattern has been shown to impose a severe stress on many systems of the body and over a period of years be a principle cause of death from heart attacks.

Research studies over the last decade have demonstrated rather convincingly that the most desirable eating habits would be those which provide an optimum amount of all nutrients to the cells at all times. This condition is achieved for the fetus via the placenta in a well-nourished woman but detoriorates throughout the life span of the child from: demand feeding, to 4 meals a day, to 3 meals a day, to 2½ meals, and sometimes to 2 very irregular meals a day.

Doctors have known for a long time that people fed small meals more frequently, respond best to treatment and this has been the feeding schedule in first-class hospitals for many years.

Consequently, there is general agreement today that the ideal meal pattern is frequent, smaller meals, each of which provides a mixture of all the nutrients. With a little planning, this can be achieved without a heavy burden being imposed on the cook, or without over-eating. Such a pattern provides for vitality throughout the day rather than the hunger — overfed — drowsy — hunger sequence associated with large infrequent meals.

3

Know Your Activity Needs

MOST OF THE food we eat is used to provide energy for our bodies. In fact, the most important function food performs in the body is to supply energy, for without energy no cell could perform its functions or long survive. Food is burned in the body somewhat like coal and oil are burned in a furnace. Just as the energy released from coal and oil is used to heat homes and drive machinery, the energy released from food heats our bodies and drives our bodily machinery. When nutrients are burned or oxidized in the cells, energy is released and made available to drive the cell's reactions. This oxidation is relatively efficient, but some of the energy is lost as heat. Although some of this heat is used to maintain body temperature, the rest of the heat is wasted energy and must be dissipated or excreted from the body because the body temperature must be maintained within relatively narrow limits. Most of this extra heat is excreted through radiation from the body surface, as hot, moist expired air and as hot urine.

Energy is typically measured as heat (heat released when the material is burned) and expressed as calories. One calorie or kilocalorie (C or Kcal.) is the amount of heat required to raise the temperature of one kilogram (2.2 lbs. or about 1 quart) of water one degree centigrade. Therefore, a calorie is not a nutrient but a unit of measure and used to express the energy value of foods or their energy containing nutrients: carbohydrates, fats, and proteins.

MEASUREMENT OF CALORIES

The energy values of foods are established by measuring the calories of heat given off when the food is ignited and burned in equipment especially designed for the purpose. The bomb calorimeter is the most widely used instrument to measure the energy value of food. A weighed sample of food is placed in the bomb, which is filled with oxygen. This bomb or container is then placed in an insulated water bath which contains a known amount of water. The food in the bomb is burned completely after an electric spark ignites the food and the heat given off will always cause the temperature of the bomb and then the surrounding water to increase a certain number of degrees per gram of that particular food. A sensitive thermometer, which can be read to a thousandth of a degree, is used to measure the temperature of the water before and after combustion. From the increase in the temperature reading, the energy value or fuel value of the food can be calculated.

The bomb calorimeter was originally used to establish the caloric values of pure fat, carbohydrate, and protein. However, it was soon discovered that several corrections were necessary when calculating the energy values of human diets, because the body was not as efficient as the calorimeter. Extensive experimentation revealed that the following figures were suitable for estimating the amount of energy supplied by various mixed diets:

1 gram of carbohydrate	=	4 calories
1 gram of fat	=	9 calories
1 gram of protein	=	4 calories

CALORIC VALUES OF COMMON FOODS

The U.S. Department of Agriculture has published extensive tables of the caloric value of hundreds of foods. Table 3-1 lists many of the common foods that are regularly eaten by athletes and college students.

ENERGY NEEDS

The total energy requirement of an individual is dependent upon the amount of energy required for maintaining basal metabolism, physical activity, sleep, growth, pregnancy, lactation, rehabilitation from disease or inactivity, the specific dynamic effect, and the maintenance of ideal body temperature.

41

TABLE 3-1
CALORIE VALUES OF COMMON FOODS

Food	Weight or approximate measure	Calories
MILK GROUP		
Cheese, cheddar	1-1/8 cube	115
Cheese, cottage, creamed	1/4 cup	65
Cream, coffee	1 tbsp	30
Milk, fluid, skim (buttermilk)	1 cup	90
Milk, fluid, whole	1 cup	160
MEAT GROUP		
Beans, dry, canned	3/4 cup	233
Beef, pot roast	3 oz.	245
Chicken	1/2 breast—with bone	155
Egg	1 medium	80
Frankfurter	1 medium	170
Haddock	1 fillet	140
Ham, boiled	2 oz.	135
Liver, beef	2 oz.	130
Peanut butter	2 tbsp	190
Pork chop	1 chop	260
Salmon, canned	1/2 cup	120
Sausage, bologna	2 slices	173
VEGETABLE GROUP		
Beans, snap, green	1/2 cup	15
Broccoli	1/2 cup	20
Cabbage, shredded, raw	1/2 cup	10
Carrots, diced	1/2 cup	23
Corn, canned	1/2 cup	85
Lettuce leaves	2 large or 4 small	10
Peas, green	1/2 cup	58
Potato, white	1 medium	90
Spinach	1/2 cup	20
Squash, winter	1/2 cup	65
Sweet potato	1 medium	155
Tomato juice, canned	1/2 cup (small glass)	23
FRUIT GROUP		
Apple, raw	1 medium	70
Apricots, dried, stewed	1/2 cup	135
Banana, raw	1 medium	100
Cantaloupe	1/2 melon	60
Grapefruit	1/2 medium	45
Orange	1 medium	65
Orange juice, fresh	1/2 cup (small glass)	55
Peaches, canned	1/2 cup with syrup	100
Pineapple juice, canned	1/2 cup (small glass)	68
Prunes, dried, cooked	5 with juice	160
Strawberries, raw	1/2 cup, capped	30
BREAD-CEREAL GROUP		
Bread, white, enriched	1 slice	70
Cornflakes, fortified	1-1/3 cup	133
Macaroni, enriched, cooked	3/4 cup	115
Oatmeal, cooked	2/3 cup	87
Rice, cooked	3/4 cup	140

FATS GROUP		
Bacon, crisp	2 slices	90
Butter or fortified margarine	1 tbsp	100
Oils, salad or cooking	1 tbsp	125
SWEETS GROUP		
Beverages, cola type	6 oz.	75
Sugar, granulated	1 tbsp	40

The basal metabolism is the minimum amount of cell reaction needed to carry on the vital or life processes of the body when it is awake. Energy required for the performance of physical activity ranks second to the amount of energy required for basal metabolism. Energy must also be supplied to meet the needs of an increasing number or activity of cells during growth, pregnancy, lactation, or rehabilitation from disease or inactivity.

The extra energy required to utilize nutrients by the cells (specific dynamic effect) is the fourth factor that is part of the total energy requirement, although this factor is relatively small compared to the first three. Finally, an amount of energy is required to maintain the ideal body temperature if the environment is very hot or cold. Under very cold conditions, the typical inefficiency and energy loss from the cell reactions is not sufficient to maintain ideal body temperature. If your clothing is unable to keep the body warmth in and the cold air out, you may begin to shiver or stamp your feet in order to generate more body warmth by causing more cells to become active. Under very hot conditions, the body may actually have to work to keep cool by increasing the rate of respiration and by profuse perspiration.

ENERGY REQUIRED FOR BASAL METABOLISM

The basal energy requirement of an individual can be determined by a respiration apparatus. This apparatus measures the oxygen used during a specific period of time ... which is dependent upon the amount of oxidation (or energy utilization) taking place in the subject.

The energy used or required affects the subject's basal or minimal metabolism if the measurement is made while the subject is: awake but completely relaxed and rested, is not under emotional stress, has fasted overnight, and if the test is conducted at a comfortable temperature and humidity. These results are expressed as calories/day and reflect the amount of energy required for maintenance of one's minimal activities.

It is also possible for you to estimate the basal energy requirement. One simple method is based on body weight as follows:

Basal Energy Requirement   =   1 cal. × body weight (kg.)
                                                    × 24 hrs. (in cal./24 hrs.)

The kilograms of body weight are found by dividing the weight in pounds by 2.2. The calculation for the energy needed for the basal metabolism of a college man weighing 187 pounds would be:

Basal Energy Requirement   =   1 × 187/2.2 × 24
                              =   2040 cal./24 hrs.

The basal metabolism or energy requirement is also affected by factors other than body weight such as body structure or composition (bone density, amount of muscle, fat, water present), age, climate, sex, general health, growth, pregnancy, and lactation.

ENERGY REQUIRED FOR PHYSICAL ACTIVITIES

Any kind of physical activity increases the energy expenditure above the basal caloric need, even if the activity is merely eating, sitting, or standing. The amount of energy needed for physical activity by the moderately-active man or woman usually comprises the second greatest caloric expenditure (second only to the basal energy requirement). However, this would not be true for a very active individual, such as a basketball player, a distance runner, or a lumberjack. In these subjects, the energy required for physical activity would probably exceed the basal energy requirement.

Several factors determine the energy cost of physical activity: the kind of activity, the intensity and duration of the activity performed, the skill of the participant, and the body size of the individual. Table 3-2 lists factors that can be used to calculate the cost of certain physical activities.

ENERGY REQUIRED FOR GROWTH, REPAIR, PREGNANCY AND LACTATION

The energy required for growth, repair, pregnancy, and lactation changes and depends upon the rate or stage of the growth

TABLE 3-2
ESTIMATION OF CALORIES FOR ACTIVITIES FOR VARIOUS TYPES OF DAYS

Type of Activity	Cal per lb per hr
A. At rest most of day (sitting, reading, etc., very little walking and standing)	0.23
B. Very light exercise (sitting most of the day, studying, with about 2 hr of walking and standing)	0.27
C. Light exercise (sitting, typing, standing, laboratory work, walking, etc.)	0.36
D. Moderate exercise (standing, walking, housework, gardening, carpentry, etc., little sitting)	0.50
E. Severe exercise (standing, walking, skating, outdoor games, dancing, etc., little sitting)	0.77
F. Very severe exercise (sports—tennis, swimming, basketball, football, running—heavy work, etc., little sitting)	1.09

process. If adequate amounts of energy sources are not provided, growth is retarded and finally all cell activity is reduced. Approximately 10 percent of the body's energy sources are used during growth or repair of tissues.

ENERGY REQUIRED FOR UTILIZING THE INGESTED FOOD

The factor next considered in estimating the daily energy requirement is the energy required to utilize the diet. This increase has been referred to as a "tax" that is added to the total calorie intake for utilizing the ingested nutrients. If the diet was exclusively one of the following foods, the tax would be: carbohydrate — 6 percent, fat — 14 percent, and protein — 30 percent of the caloric value of that food. Since most people eat a mixed diet, the average energy increase is estimated to be less than 10 percent. By adding together the calories for basal metabolism and physical activities and taking 10 percent of this total, the energy required to digest, absorb and metabolize food can be estimated. In this way the total amount of energy required by an individual can be determined. Table 3-3 shows an example of such combined estimations.

TABLE 3-3
SHORT-CUT METHOD OF ESTIMATING YOUR
DAILY CALORIE NEED

A. Weigh yourself; using your body weight as a basis, estimate your basal calorie need for 24 hours.

B. Keep a diary of your activities for a typical day. Decide from Table 3-2 in which category you belong: A, B, C, D, E, or F. Calculate the calorie need for your activities, for one day.

C. Total your calorie needs, taking into consideration the 10 percent "tax" for influence of food.

Sample of Calculation:

Assume: an adult weighing 125 lbs (57 kg)
a day with 16 hr of activity; 8 hr of sleep
category of activity: C, light exercise

1. Calories for basal metabolism (corrected for saving in sleep)
Basal metabolism for 24 hr — 1368 cal (1 x 57 x 24)
Saving in sleep, 8 hr — − 46 cal (0.1 x 57 x 8)
1322

2. Add calories for activity (0.36 x 125 x 16) = 720; 1322 + 720 = 2042

3. Add calories for the influence of food (10 percent of 2042) = 204

4. Total estimated calories needed for the day (2042 + 204) = 2246

SPORTS WITH SMALL ENERGY COSTS

Many sports are single efforts, such as the shot put, discus, diving, and ski jumping. Others are of short duration, such as short-distance skiing and swimming, sprinting, and hurdling. Although these events require strength and ability to react quickly, your energy needs are increased relatively little if these sports are practiced less than an hour a day. Additional sports that require relatively small amounts of energy expenditure are listed below:

Archery	High jump
Baseball	Hurdle races
Boating	Javelin throw
Bowling	Pole vaulting
Canoeing, slow or moderate speed	Rowing, slow or moderate speed
Cycling, slow or moderate speed	Shooting
Dancing	Short-distance running
Diving	Short-distance skiing
Equestrian sports	Short-distance swimming
Fencing	Shot put
Golf	Skating
	Ski jumping

| Softball | Volleyball |
| Tennis | Weightlifting |

SPORTS WITH LARGE ENERGY COSTS

Sports requiring extra energy expenditure over long periods of time are listed here. Preseason conditioning and the hours of training required in sports such as swimming, track, football, and basketball may increase the total caloric needs to as high as 4,000 to 5,000 calories per day, depending on body size and weight. A list of sports which require relatively large amounts of any expenditure are as follows:

Basketball	Long-distance skiing
Boxing	Long-distance swimming
Football	Marathon
Gymnastics (especially apparatus)	Middle-distance running
	Mountaineering
Handball	Paddleball
Hockey (ice and field)	Pantathlon
	Skindiving
Judo	Squash
Long-distance canoeing	Soccer
Long-distance rowing	Tumbling
Long-distance running	Water Polo
Long-distance skating	Wrestling

Almost any sport with relatively low-energy cost can be placed in the high-energy classification if it is carried on intensively for a long time. For example, the prolonged golf game or tennis match could also fall into this category.

GUIDELINES FOR A NUTRITIONALLY SOUND DIET

The first step for the athlete in developing a sound diet is to determine his present dietary habits. On the following pages, several ways in which you can evaluate your current eating habits are described.

1. Select a day that is representative of your eating habits (usually a week day).
2. Write down what you eat at each meal and between meals.
3. Record food quantities in the food groups column.

For example, if you ate the following for breakfast:

½ cup orange juice
1 egg
2 slices of buttered toast
1 cup milk

you would record it as follows:

	Milk Group	Meat Group	Fruits and Vegetables	Bread and Cereal	Additional Foods
Breakfast	1	1	1	2	2

Record the other foods consumed throughout the day in a similar manner on the "Typical One Day Meal Record" table and then transfer these total amounts to the "Food Scoreboard" that applies most nearly to your daily energy requirements.

TYPICAL ONE DAY MEAL RECORD

Food Groups

Meal	Milk Group (cups)	Meat Group (servings)	Fruits and Vegetables (servings)	Bread and Cereal (servings)	Additional Foods like fats, candy desserts, soft drinks, snacks
Breakfast					
Mid-morning snack					
Lunch					
Afternoon snack					
Dinner					

**Evening
snack**

===

TOTALS

_____

FOOD SCOREBOARD (Approximately 2,500 calories)

Recommended Food	Goal	Score
Milk	3 cups	_____
Meat	5 ounces	_____
Fruits and Vegetables	8 servings	_____
Fruits	6 servings	_____
Vegetables	2 servings	_____
Bread	8 servings	_____
	4 with jelly	_____
Other	2 desserts	_____
	2 teaspoons oil	_____

Take a look at your score. You may find that you have been leaving out important foods, and if so, you need to start including them. Or you may find that you have been eating too many "empty" calories such as carbonated beverages and candy.

Foods to Add

_____

_____

_____

Foods to Cut Down On

_____

_____

_____

FOOD SCOREBOARD (Approximately 3,750 calories)

Recommended Food	Goal	Score
Milk	4½ cups	_____
Meat	7½ ounces	_____
Fruits and Vegetables	12 servings	_____
Fruits	9 servings	_____
Vegetables	3 servings	_____

Bread	12 servings	_____
	6 with jelly	_____
Other	3 desserts and	_____
	3 teaspoons oil	_____

Take a look at your score. You may find that you have been leaving out important foods, and if so, you need to start including them. Or you may find that you have been eating too many "empty" calories such as carbonated beverages and candy.

Foods to Add   **Foods to Cut Down On**

_____   _____
_____   _____
_____   _____

FOOD SCOREBOARD (Approximate by 5,000 calories)

Recommended Foods	Goal	Score
Milk	6 cups	_____
Meat	10 ounces	_____
Fruits and Vegetables	16 servings	_____
Fruits	12 servings	_____
Vegetables	4 servings	_____
Bread	16 servings	_____
	8 with jelly	_____
Other	4 desserts	_____
	4 teaspoons oil	_____

Take a look at your score. You may find that you have been leaving out important foods, and if so, you need to start including them. Or you may find that you have been eating too many "empty" calories such as carbonated beverages and candy.

Foods to Add   **Foods to Cut Down On**

_____   _____
_____   _____
_____   _____

These food scoreboards were developed according to the basic diet described by the Food and Nutrition Board of the National

Research Council. This diet consists of two to four cups of milk a day, two servings of meat, four or more servings of fruits and vegetables, and four or more servings from the bread group. By following this procedure you will be able to test the nutritional quality or adequacy of your diet.

Recent research shows that the average American consumes over 3,400 calories a day. Of these calories, 45 percent comes from carbohydrates, 12 percent from proteins, and 43 percent from fat food sources. Nutrition and medical authorities are in agreement that Americans consume too many calories. These calories are provided primarily by refined sugars and fat.

Americans consume many pastries and other desserts, foods fried in fat, and a lot of beef. The average American eats over 100 grams of protein each day primarily in the form of meat and dairy products. Although these foods contain high quality protein, amounts eaten in excess of body needs are converted to fat. They furthermore contain an appreciable amount of fat, which is the most concentrated form of energy in the diet.

Authorities also recommend that the fat content of the American diet should be reduced to approximately 30-35 percent. Therefore the optimum diet for health should look like this as far as proportions are concerned:

	Fat	Protein	Carbo-hydrate
Average American Diet	43%	12%	45%
Optimum Diet for Health	30-35%	12-15%	55-58%

Using these guidelines I've developed diets for three energy levels: diets which provide 2,500, 3,750, and 5,000 calories per day. The diets are described by listing the appropriate amounts of the food groups, as well as their nutrient content.

TOTAL SERVINGS OF FOODS IN DAILY MEAL SCHEDULES

Approximate Calories	Whole Milk	Meat or Equivalent	Fruit	Veg.	Bread	Other
2,500	3 cups	5 ounces	6 ser.	2 ser.	8 ser. 4 with jelly	2 desserts 2 tsp. oil
3,750	4½ cups	7½ ounces	9 ser.	3 ser.	12 ser. 6 with jelly	3 desserts 3 tsp. oil
5,000	6 cups	10 ounces	12 ser.	4 ser.	16 ser. 8 with jelly	4 desserts 4 tsp. oil

APPROXIMATE NUTRIENT CONTENT OF DAILY MEAL SCHEDULE

Approximate Calories	FAT		PROTEIN		CARBOHYDRATE	
	Grams	% Total Calories	Grams	% Total Calories	Grams	% Total Calories
2,500	70	28	79	13	374	59
3,750	105	28	118	13	561	59
5,000	140	28	158	13	748	59

You will notice that the nutrient content of these daily schedules is almost the same as the "Optimum Diet for Health." I have added an extra percentage point for the athlete in protein and carbohydrate foods and deducted two from the fat sources. I believe this will benefit the athlete's performance.

The daily meal schedules were developed for three energy levels: 2,500, 3,750, and 5,000 calories. From these three diets, you should be able to plan your own special diet. For example, the 135-pound golfer might require 2,500 calories a day, as well as the 110-pound female gymnast. On the other hand, the 225 pound football player should probably consume close to 5,000 calories as should the 165-pound swimmer in rigorous training. And in between these athletes is the 175-pound weightlifter-bodybuilder who would require around 3,750 calories per day.

Perhaps you are thinking that it might be difficult to consume 5,000 calories a day, and it would if you stuck to three meals a day. The listing here indicates how 5,000 calories can be consumed by eating three meals as well as three snacks each day. Of course, this sample diet is only offered as a guideline. You may want to substitute ice cream, fruit juice, popcorn, or cookies in the snack area. There are many foods that can be substituted for those listed.

EXAMPLE MEAL SCHEDULE FOR 5,000 CALORIES

1. Breakfast
     2 cups milk
     3 ounces meat
     2 servings of fruit

2 servings of bread
2 servings of bread with jelly
2. Mid-morning snack
2 servings of fruit
2 servings of bread with jelly
3. Lunch
2 cups milk
3 ounces meat
2 servings of fruit
2 servings of vegetables
3 servings of bread
2 desserts
2 teaspoon oil
4. Afternoon snack
2 servings of fruit
2 servings of bread with jelly
5. Dinner
2 cups milk
4 ounces meat
2 servings of fruit
2 servings of vegetables
3 servings of bread
2 desserts
2 teaspoon oil
6. Evening snack
2 servings of fruit
2 servings of bread with jelly

QUESTIONS AND ANSWERS

Question: **What is an average serving?**
Answer: An average serving can be defined in numerous ways. A serving of mashed potatoes is about the same size as a large scoop or one serving of ice cream. A serving of meat is usually considered to be three ounces, a serving of orange juice is about three ounces or half a cup, and a serving of apple pie is 1/6 of a 9-inch pie. In addition, a serving of egg is the whole thing, a serving of bread is one slice, and a serving of cereal is ¾ cup.

Question: **How accurate are "calorie tables?"**
Answer: Calorie tables are estimates at best. Numerous fac-

tors affect the accuracy of the estimates, the most important of which is the variation in food composition.

Calories are an expression or measure of the energy that can be derived from food. The major energy-providing nutrients are carbohydrates, fats, and proteins. The energy available in a food can be measured by combustion of the food in a calorimeter or it can be estimated arithmetically by calculation, for example (grams of carbohydrates in the diet × 4 cal) + (grams of fat in the diet × 9 cal) + (grams of protein in the diet × 4 cal). Although conventional food composition tables are carefully done and based on averages of many analyses they must be used with discretion because of the variation in the composition of foods, variable effects of cooking, storage, stage of ripeness, quality of the food, etc.

Question: **What would a sample meal schedule for an athlete look like on paper?**

Answer: Two meal sample schedules for athletes are listed below.

TWO SAMPLE MEAL SCHEDULES (approximately 2,700 calories)

FOOD LIST CHOICES		FOOD LIST CHOICES	
BREAKFAST		**BREAKFAST**	
Milk*	1 cup	Milk*	1 cup cocoa
Citrus fruit	1/2 grapefruit	Citrus fruit	1/2 cup orange juice
Enriched Bread (2 servings)	1 cup oatmeal	Meat equivalent	1 poached egg
Enriched Bread (4 servings)	2 sweet rolls	Enriched bread	3 slices toast
Butter or margarine	3 tsp.	Butter or margarine	3 tsp.
LUNCH		**LUNCH**	
Meat or equivalents (2 servings)	2 slices cheese	Meat or equivalent (1 serving)	2 tbsp. peanut butter
Bread and substitute (3 servings)	1 bun & potato chips (1 oz. bag)	Enriched bread	2 slices
Vegetables	Lettuce and tomato (for sandwich) Celery sticks	Butter or margarine	1 tsp.
		Bread substitute (1 serving)	5 crackers
Milk*	1 cup	Vegetables	Vegetable soup
		Bread substitute (2 servings)	Pound cake (small slice)
		Milk*	1 cup
AFTERNOON SNACK		**AFTERNOON SNACK**	
Fruit	Fruit in season	Bread substitute (2 servings) and	
Bread substitute** (3 servings)	Cup cake	fat substitute (2 servings)	1 cup ice cream
DINNER		**DINNER**	
Meat or equivalent (3 servings)	Meat loaf (5 oz.)***	Meat (3 oz.)	Pork chop, lean (no bone)
Bread substitute (2 servings)	Baked potato	Bread substitute (2 servings)	1 cup noodles
Vegetables	Broccoli Salad	Vegetables	Peas and carrots Salad

Dressing	2 tsp.		Dressing	2 tsp.
(fat substitute)			(fat substitute)	
Enriched bread	2 rolls		Enriched bread	2 slices
(2 servings)			Butter or margarine	2 tsp.
Butter or margarine	4 tsp.		Fruit	Fruit in season
Fruit	Fruit in season		Plain dessert	2 cookies
Milk*	1 cup		Milk*	1 cup

EVENING SNACK			EVENING SNACK	
Chocolate milk	1 cup		Milk*	1 cup milk
Simple dessert	1 tbsp. chocolate sauce		Bread equivalent	2 cups popcorn
			(2 servings)	

*Milk-- Low fat (2% butter fat)
**A calorie equivalent but not in nutrient content.
***Meat loaf has bread crumbs and some filler, so extra weight is allowed.

TWO SAMPLE MEAL SCHEDULES (approximately 3,000 calories)

FOOD LIST CHOICES

BREAKFAST

Citrus fruit	1/2 grapefruit
Bread substitute	1 cup oatmeal
(2 servings)	
Enriched bread	2 slices toast
Butter or margarine	2 tsp.
Jelly or sugar	1 tbsp.
Milk*	1 cup

LUNCH

Meat equivalents (4)	Cheeseburger
	3 oz. beef
	1 slice cheese
Bread substitutes	1 bun & potato
(4 servings)	chips (2 oz. bag)
Vegetables	Onion
	(for cheeseburger)
	Carrot sticks
Plain dessert	Cookie (3")
Milk*	1 cup

AFTERNOON SNACK

Fruit	Fruit in season
Bread substitute	2 cups popcorn
(2 servings)	

DINNER

Meat (3 oz.)	Meat loaf (5 oz.)**
Bread substitute	Baked potato
(2 servings)	
	Broccoli
	Salad
Dressing	2 tsp.
Enriched bread	2 rolls
Butter or margarine	4 tsp.
Fruit	Fruit in season
Milk*	1 cup
Bread substitute	Plain cake
(2 servings)	

EVENING SNACK

Milk*	1 cup
Bread substitute	
(1 serving and	
fat substitute)	} 1/2 cup ice cream
(1 serving)	
Plain dessert	1 tbsp. sauce

FOOD LIST CHOICES

BREAKFAST

Citrus fruit	1 cup tomato juice
Meat equivalent	1 poached egg
Enriched bread	3 slices toast
Butter or margarine	2 tsp.
Milk*	1 cup cocoa

LUNCH

Meat equivalents (2)	1 slice cheese
	2 tbsp. peanut butter
Enriched bread	3 slices
Butter or margarine	2 tsp.
Bread substitute	5 crackers
(1 serving)	
Vegetables	Vegetable soup
Plain dessert	Cupcake
(2 servings)	

AFTERNOON SNACK

Bread substitute	3 cookies (3")
(3 servings)	

DINNER

Meat (4 oz.)	2 pork chops, lean
	(no bone)
Bread substitute	1 cup noodles
(2 servings)	
Vegetables	Peas and carrots
	Salad
Dressing	2 tsp.
(fat substitute)	
Butter or margarine	2 tsp.
Enriched bread	2 slices
Fruit	Apricot halves
Bread substitute	2 cookies (3")
(2 servings)	

EVENING SNACK

Milk*	1 cup
Bread substitute	2 cups popcorn
(2 servings)	

*Milk—Low fat (2% butter fat)
**Meat loaf has bread crumbs and some filler, so extra weight is allowed.

55

Question: **Should the athlete eat between meals?**

Answer: Eating between meals isn't necessarily bad, in fact, it may actually be the most desirable eating pattern, if it does not unbalance the day's total nutrient intake, especially of calories. All between meal snacks must be counted when calculating the total scores of your one-day meal record and the food scoreboard. The goal is to satisfy the subject's nutrient requirements each day, or better yet, a balanced proportion of them at each meal or snack. A snack list, with approximate calories included, is shown below.

SNACK AND DESSERT LIST*

	Approximate Calories
Milk shake (fountain size)	400
Malted milk shake (fountain size)	500
Sundaes	215-325
Sodas	260
Hamburger (including bun)	360
Hot dog (including bun)	210
Pizza (4"-5" section)	135
Popcorn, lightly buttered (½ cup)	75
Nuts (3 tbsp. chopped, or 30 peanuts)	150
Pound cake (3/8" slice)	140
Cup cake with frosting (2-3/4" diam.)	185
Layer cake with frosting (2" slice)	370-445
Pancake (4" diam.)	60
Waffle (medium, 4½" x 5½" x ½")	215
Add 20 calories for each teaspoon syrup or sweetening	
Add 45 calories for each teaspoon butter or other fat spread	
Brownies (2" x 2" x ¾")	140
Plain cookie (3" diam.)	120
Pie (1/8 of a 9" pie)	275-345
Fruit juice (1 cup)	110-165

*One slice of bread is approximately 70 calories. When these foods are used in place of bread they will not have the same nutritive value.

Question: **What is the opinion of health authorities on the sale of candy and soft drinks in schools?**

Answer: The Council on Foods and Nutrition of the American Medical Association recently published the following statement:

> One of the functions of a school lunch program is to provide training in sound food habits. The sale of foods, confections, and beverages in lunchrooms, recreation

rooms, and other school facilities influences directly the food habits of the students. Every effort should be extended to encourage students to adopt and enjoy good food habits. The availability of confections and carbonated beverages on school premises may tempt children to spend lunch money for them and lead to poor food habits.

Soft drinks and many snack foods provide no nutrients other than calories and therefore tend to unbalance the diet as well as reduce the child's appetite for regular meals.

Expenditures for carbonated beverages and most confections yield a nutritional return greatly inferior to that of milk, fruit, and other foods included in the basic food groups. When given a choice between carbonated beverages and milk, or between candy and fruit, a child may choose the less nutritious. In view of these considerations, the Council on Foods and Nutrition is particularly opposed to the sale and distribution of confections and carbonated beverages in school lunchrooms.

Question: **Is food obtained from vending machines always safe to eat?**

Answer: In recent years, there has been a phenomenal growth in the food vending industry. It is now possible to get a complete meal. At one time, the only food items associated with the vending machines were gum, candy, and similar nonperishable items. But now, vending machines distribute potentially hazardous foods. For example, milk, eggs, and meat are capable of supporting rapid growth of infectious or toxin-producing micro-organisms. Not only must these foods be prepared under sanitary conditions, but they must be transported in refrigerated vehicles and dispensed in refrigerated vending machines. The foods must be replaced frequently in the vending machines and discarded should a power failure occur. A machine with slow turnover in an out-of-the-way location may contain spoiled foods, especially if the wrapper has been broken.

Generally speaking, the food-vending industry has made great strides in ensuring that its new products are fit to eat, but breaks in the merchandising chain do occur occasionally. Regulations for the sale of such foods were prepared through the cooperative efforts of the National Automatic Merchandising Association, the U.S. Public Health Service, and the state and local health agencies.

Question: **What is an athlete's basal metabolic requirement, and how does this relate to his total caloric requirement?**

Answer: An athlete's basal requirement refers to the calories he needs to maintain his involuntary body functions and proper body temperature. In other words, it is his minimum cost of living.

A male athlete, 18 years old, five feet ten inches tall, weighing 175 pounds, has a basal metabolic requirement of about 1,800 calories. His recommended (total) caloric intake for moderate activity and two hours of training, is 3,000 calories per day. The difference of 1,200 calories, between his basal metabolic requirement and recommended caloric intake represents the number of calories he expends for voluntary activities. In one sense, it is his "energy checking account." If all 1,200 calories aren't used during the day's activity, those remaining are transferred from the "checking account" to a "savings account" and thus accumulate in the form of fat. On the other hand, if the athlete overdraws his checking account, the savings are called on and fat loss results. Therefore, a relatively small "energy savings account" in the form of body fat is usually desirable.

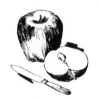

4

Fill'er Up With Energy

WHAT TYPES of foods do athletes prefer for energy? A survey taken at the Munich Olympics revealed a wide variety of choices. Olga Connolly, former Olympic champion in the women's discus, commented, "I just love whipping cream as an energy food." Whipping cream is noted for its high-fat content. In similar fashion, Russ Knipp of the U.S. weightlifting team and former National champion in the middleweight class is a strong believer in wheat germ oil as an energy food. He said, "I can definitely feel a lag in my endurance when I quit taking wheat germ oil."

However, there are many athletes that avoid eating fat-containing foods during their training programs. An example of this attitude is the statement by Kathy Hammond, bronze medal winner in the women's 400-meter run. Kathy stated, "I avoid eating most types of fatty foods in my training, especially in the meal preceding my competition."

Jack Bacheler, Olympic marathoner and 1969 AAU Cross-Country champion made the following remarks concerning energy foods in his diet:

> I've gotten good results from eating a high-carbohydrate diet several days prior to my competition. I will also drink 64 ounces of uncarbonated Coke (8, 8-ounce plastic bottles) at intervals along the way during my marathon running. This seems to give me an additional kick.

On the other hand, Ray Seales of the U.S. boxing team and Olympic champion in the light welterweight class avoids many carbohydrate foods in his training. He remarked, "I don't eat any bread or starch. It makes me soft inside." And then there is the statement of sprinters Eddie Hart and Robert Taylor of the gold medal winning 400-meter relay, "We don't eat any special foods for energy. We just get out there and run!"

It is obvious from the above remarks that Olympic athletes hold different ideas concerning food and energy sources. Which of these concepts are actually valid or supported by scientific evidence and which are not? After reading this chapter you should be able to select appropriate energy sources for your particular athletic event. In order to do this, it is important that you understand something about how your body unlocks and releases the potential energy of the ingested food and uses it to carry out all of the body's functions and activities.

OCCURRENCE OF CARBOHYDRATES IN FOODS

There are more carbohydrates in nature than all other organic materials combined. This is because all plants are composed primarily of carbohydrates. The plant's supporting structure (cellulose) and its storage form of energy (starch) are carbohydrates.

Plants are able to synthesize carbohydrates, fats, proteins, and vitamins from water, soil minerals, and carbon dioxide using the energy from the sun by a process called photosynthesis. However, many of the nutrients required by man must be obtained by way of the diet (secondhand from plants or third-hand from other animals that have consumed plants).

Therefore, we can speak of energy conversion rates and efficiencies. Plants convert energy much more efficiently per acre than animals, and therefore plant foods are less expensive. Although the carbohydrates, fats, minerals and vitamins are of high quality, the protein synthesized by plants is not ideally suited for man and is therefore considered to be of poor quality.

Cellulose, which is the plant's supporting structure, is the grazing animal's most important dietary carbohydrate. Man is not able to digest cellulose and therefore is unable to derive energy from this carbohydrate. Starch, which is the plant's storage form of energy, is man's most common form of dietary carbohydrate. It supplies over half of the energy sources in the American diet.

Common dietary carbohydrates are starch, from plants; table sugar or sucrose, which is refined, or pure sugar prepared from sugar cane or sugar beets; milk sugar or lactose, which is synthesized in the mammary gland; malt sugar or maltose prepared from various plants; glucose or dextrose, which is found in many fruits; and cellulose. Glucose is the carbohydrate that circulates in the blood ("blood sugar") and enters cells as one of its energy sources. Although cellulose or fiber does not provide energy for man, it is a useful dietary constituent because it supplies most of the bulk in the diet. Bulk aids in intestinal function and regularity of bowel movements (fecal excretion).

Glycogen is man's storage form of carbohydrate and is found in muscle and liver. When these storage sites are filled, any additional or extra amounts of carbohydrate consumed in the diet are converted into fat and stored as such. The body can store an almost unlimited amount of energy as fat or 100 times more energy in the form of fat than it can in the form of carbohydrate (glycogen).

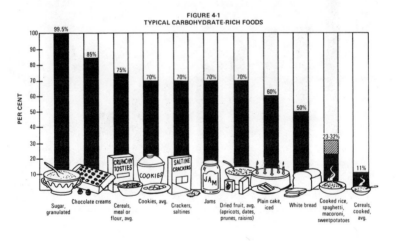

FIGURE 4-1
TYPICAL CARBOHYDRATE-RICH FOODS

In recent years, people in the United States have tended to eat less of the natural grain products and have placed more emphasis on refined sugar products such as candies and sweets. In 1970, according to the U.S. Department of Agriculture, 46 percent of the total calories were derived from carbohydrates.

OCCURRENCE OF FATS IN THE DIET
Fats include a group of rather dissimilar compounds that have been grouped together on the basis of their solubility. They

61

will not dissolve in water, but they will dissolve in fat solvents such as ether or gasoline.

Fats are found in all plant and animal tissues. Whereas plants store most of their energy as carbohydrates, man stores most of his as fats.

The chief sources of fat in the typical American diet are milk, butter, cheese, margarine, meat, fish, and cooking oils. Most people are conscious of ingesting fat when they eat butter or margarine or the visible fat with meat, however, they are not conscious of the "invisible" fat. Average lean beef will contain about eight percent or more of invisible fat. In fact, the choice grades of meat contain more fat or marbling than the poorer grades. Foods such as vegetable oils and lard are 100 percent fat, while most fruits and vegetables contain less than one percent fat. Figure 4-2 shows the fat content of some common foods.

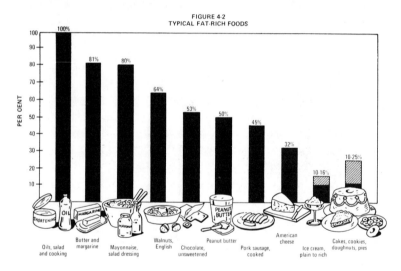

FIGURE 4-2
TYPICAL FAT-RICH FOODS

FUNCTIONS OF CARBOHYDRATES

The main function that dietary carbohydrates serve in the body is the provision of energy. Since other nutrients can also provide energy, health may be maintained on diets which differ greatly in their carbohydrate content. Some people survive on diets made up almost entirely of protein and fats, while other people live on diets that are over 80 percent carbohydrate. Carbohydrate intake is influenced primarily by economic factors. Lower income families tend to consume more carbohydrates, and higher income families consume more proteins and fats. On the average, carbohydrate consumption has decreased in the United States since 1900.

While life can be maintained with little carbohydrate material in the diet, there is considerable evidence that a liberal intake of carbohydrate is advisable. Presumably, this is due more to the dangers or toxicity of high-fat diets and less to the special merits of dietary carbohydrates. An energy source is obviously required in the diet and there are three possible choices: carbohydrates, fats, or proteins. Carbohydrates present in various fruits are the preferred sources of energy by the body since they are easily absorbed and require less alternation prior to the release of their energy. If the dietary source for energy is one other than protein, then the expensive proteins can be used more appropriately as building blocks and will not have to be burned to supply energy.

Since too many saturated fats in the diet have been shown to be linked to cardiovascular disease, they must be kept at a reasonable level. But saturated fats are a useful and desirable component in the diet if they are consumed in moderation and balanced with the amount of polyunsaturated fats in the diet.

So a mixture of approximately 2 to 1 of carbohydrates to fats, with an emphasis on the polyunsaturated fats, seems to be the desirable energy source. Protein is a very important dietary constituent, but it will not be used efficiently or as it should be without a non-protein energy source in the diet.

In summary, the main contributions of carbohydrate-rich foods are to:

1. Provide an economical energy supply.
2. Furnish some proteins, minerals, and vitamins (whole grains, legumes, and potatoes).
3. Add flavor (sugar) to foods and beverages.

FUNCTIONS OF FATS

As mentioned previously, one of the signs of an affluent society is a poor diet. The diet in America is becoming increasingly rich in carbohydrates and saturated fats. Whenever people have enough money, they seem to eat a lot of meat. Most of this meat contains considerable amounts of fat or picks up considerable amounts of fat during the cooking procedure (fried in deep fat). It is estimated that Americans now consume sufficient fat to

63

provide from 40 to 45 percent of the total calories.

There are several reasons why the daily food supply should contain fat, but not as much as is currently consumed in prosperous countries. There is considerable evidence to show that people who consume large amounts of fat have the greatest incidence of death due to cardiovascular or heart disease. However, in moderation, dietary fats do perform several useful functions:

1. As a source of essential fatty acid.
2. As carriers of fat-soluble vitamins A, D, E, and K.
3. As a concentrated source of energy.
4. For making foods appetizing.
5. For satiety value.

QUESTIONS AND ANSWERS CONCERNING ENERGY AND ATHLETIC PERFORMANCE

Question: **What are the best "quick energy" or precontest foods for the athlete?**

Answer: A study was reported by Dr. Dale O. Nelson of Utah State University in *Scholastic Coach* which indicates how some coaches responded to this question. Nelson surveyed the dietary beliefs of various athletic coaches and noted that the following foods were thought to be the best quick energy sources or precontest meals for competing athletes: oranges, dextrose or glucose, honey, vitamin C tablets, chocolate, Coke, and sugar. These foods are composed mainly of carbohydrates (with the exception of vitamin C and chocolate) and are good energy sources. Although some of the coaches and athletes who use these products claim they provide almost immediate surges of energy, research in this area indicates that only athletes who compete in long endurance-type contests (e.g. marathon running and skiing) are benefitted by the use of certain high-carbohydrate diets. Dr. Peter V. Karpovich, prominent physiologist at Springfield College, and Dr. P. Astrand of Sweden believe that most sports are of such short duration that there is no apparent physiological benefit from precontest meals. The energy used in competition ordinarily comes from food consumed from several days to two weeks prior to the game or contest.

Question: **Which nutrient does the body prefer for energy in athletic performance?**

Answer: The body prefers carbohydrates and fats as sources of energy rather than proteins. Early experiments suggested that the intensity or work affected whether the body preferred fat or carbohydrate to satisfy its energy requirement. The body's preference for carbohydrates or fats as energy sources is about the same during mild exercise as at rest. However, as the athlete's activity increases to his maximum, the more important the carbohydrate sources become, until finally all the energy is derived from carbohydrates. Therefore, the preference for dietary carbohydrates depends on the intensity of activity on the oxygen supply to the working muscles: the more inadequate the oxygen supply, the greater the carbohydrate utilization.

Two members of the American track and field team that competed in the Olympics (1972) in Munich made good use of this principle. Gold medal winner in the marathon, Frank Shorter, and Jack Bacheler, who finished ninth, both adhered to carbohydrate-rich diets for several days prior to the race. Shorter even gained several pounds in the process, which he considered to be an advantage in such a gruelling test of endurance. After the event both remarked how surprised they were at the amount of energy they had during the race (see p. 166).

Question: **How does the diet affect work metabolism for the athlete?**

Answer: This question has recently been investigated by a group of Swedish physiologists, directed by Dr. Jonas Bergstrom. The amount of muscle glycogen in the quadriceps femoris muscle was monitored in men during heavy exercise and with various diets. Subjects were fed for three days on one of three diets, each providing 2,800 calories: (1) a typical mixed diet; (2) a diet containing protein and fats; and (3) a diet containing carbohydrates. After the subjects received one of the diets for three days, they were subjected to maximal work time with a workload demanding 75 percent of maximal aerobic power. The subjects consuming the carbohydrate diet were able to perform for 167 minutes; the subjects consuming the typical mixed diet tolerated the workload for 114 minutes; and the subjects consuming the protein-fat diet tolerated the workload for 57 minutes.

A similar study was reported by this same research group

working in St. Erik's Hospital, Stockholm, Sweden. Two subjects exercised on a bicycle ergometer, using only one leg, while the other leg was resting. After several hours of work, the glycogen content was analyzed in each leg, showing the exercised leg being emptied while the resting leg still had normal glycogen content. For the next three days the subjects consumed a diet composed mainly of carbohydrates. Although the glycogen content of the resting leg did not increase, the glycogen content of the exercising leg was over twice as high as the rested leg. These workers concluded that different diets as well as activity have a marked influence on the capacity of the muscles to recover from activity and to store energy.

It would appear from recent research concerning the metabolism of fats and carbohydrates, that several guidelines can be offered to athletes. It has been demonstrated that the *diet* as well as *activity* can markedly influence the metabolism of fat and carbohydrate. On an adequate or balanced diet, the greater the exercise, the greater is the relative energy yield from carbohydrate. Athletes should be aware that a high-carbohydrate diet improves the capacity for prolonged intensive exercise.

Question: **Are the terms "starch" and "carbohydrates" synonymous? Are starches digestible?**

Answer: These terms are not synonymous. Starches are carbohydrates, but not all carbohydrates are starches. Carbohydrate is a general term used to identify one of the basic classes of food components. Proteins, fats, vitamins, and minerals are other such general terms. Carbohydrates can be divided into two classes: (1) simple sugars, such as glucose or dextrose (monosaccharides) and common table sugar (disaccharides); and (2) the complex carbohydrates, such as starch and cellulose (polysaccharides).

Starch is the storage form of sugar and man's principle dietary carbohydrate. Fruits and their degree of sweetness depends on the kind and amount of simple sugars produced when starch is broken down by the ripening or by cooking.

In man, the energy from starch can be utilized only after it is broken down to simple sugar by digestive enzymes. The enzyme that is most important in the digestion of starch is amylase. It is secreted by the mouth and by the pancreas, so starch digestion begins in the mouth, continues to a small extent in the stomach and is completed in the small intestine. Since the digestive enzymes in saliva are thoroughly mixed with food by chewing and since digestive enzymes can operate best on small particles of food, food should be well chewed before swallowing in order to provide for its maximum digestion and therefore maximum absorption.

Question: **Is there any food value in table sugar?**

Answer: White table sugar is a potent energy source (calories), but contains no other nutrients. Consequently, excessive amounts of sugar foods tend to unbalance the diet in the direction of calories. Foods that supply various nutrients as well as energy are much more preferred as energy sources. Dark brown sugar and molasses contain a very small amount of a number of minerals, mainly iron and calcium, and several of the B vitamins. Many times sugar improves the flavor of various foods and beverages and permits us to enjoy foods that would be fairly unpalatable. Without sugar, tart berries and fruits, ice cream, cakes, and cookies would lack flavor, while baked products would lack their light brown crust. Sugar also can serve as a good preservative when used in jams, jellies, and candied fruits.

Question: **Honey is frequently consumed in large amounts by athletes prior to competition. Are there any special ingredients in honey that make it a good quick energy food?**

Answer: Honey contains two sugars, glucose and fructose. These are the same simple sugars that are present in table sugar or sucrose and result from its digestion. Both honey and table sugar are quickly digested, and their glucose is available to the body for use. However, honey is not significantly superior to other common sweets. Unfortunately, dietary quacks have falsely promoted honey as a sweet which they say is better tolerated than other sugars. This is not true.

Taken in large quantities, honey can produce several detrimental effects. Excess amounts of honey, glucose or dextrose pills, cubes of sugar or other similar sweets tend to draw fluid from other parts of the body into the gastrointestinal tract. This shift in fluids may add to the problem of dehydration in endurance-type sports, where sweat loss can affect performance. The body also may rebel if the sugar intake is too high. A concentrated sugar solution may cause extra distention in the stomach, and evacuation mechanisms may be impaired. Problems such as cramps, nausea, diarrhea can occur. Therefore, no more than 50 grams of a sugar (3 rounded tablespoons) in a liquid should be taken during any one-hour lapse. And even then, these foods do not seem to improve performance in short-term events.

Question: **What's the difference between fats, carbohydrates, and proteins?**

Answer: There are essentially three kinds of foods that your body uses for fuel or maintenance (building and replacing cells).

Protein, from the flesh of animals, poultry, fish, from dairy products, eggs, and from nuts and some grains.

Fats, from meat, oils, nuts and grains, and milk products.

Carbohydrates, the starches and sugars in fruits and vegetables, and in bread, pastries, and everything else made with flour and/or sugar. (Other nutrients in foods that do not supply energy, but are necessary are the many vitamins and minerals.)

These three types of foods, while being distinct, are still chemical cousins. For example, all three have a chemical spine that is composed of carbon atoms, with arms of hydrogen and oxygen. But proteins are far more complex than carbohydrates and fats. Proteins also contain nitrogen, and sometimes sulfur. Fats, however, have far less oxygen and thus contain more calories than proteins or carbohydrates. Carbohydrates, on the other hand, are the easiest of the food substances to digest.

Question: **Should the athlete restrict his consumption of fats, fried foods, and oily dressings?**

Answer: The human body needs a certain amount of fat for proper functioning. Fats in the diet are carriers of the fat-soluble vitamins A, D, E, and K; and one fatty acid, linoleic. These are essential nutrients. Furthermore, fat provides flavor, satisfaction, variety, and a concentrated form of energy. When fats enter the intestinal tract, they cause the release of a hormone, enterogastrone, which slows down the emptying time of the stomach. Although this provides a longer period of satiety (satisfaction) after a meal, there are times when slow stomach emptying may be undesirable and fat intake should be limited, such as the pregame meal.

Most fats are digested at about the same rate whether they are in the form of butter, margarine, salad dressings, shortening, or the natural fat content of food. The normal athlete can successfully digest food fried in fat that has not been burned or that does not contain other contaminants. Therefore, moderate amounts of fried foods are not taboo for the athlete.

Question: **Much confusion exists around the word cholesterol and such adjectives as saturated, unsaturated, polyunsaturated, hydrogenated, and partially hydrogenated when applied to salad oils, cooking oils, margarines, and shortening. What do they all mean?**

Answer: Cholesterol is a fat that animal cells (including man) can synthesize from building blocks provided by the breakdown of dietary carbohydrates and fats. It is made and used by most cells in the body and is required for optimal health. Cholesterol is not found in plants.

Saturated fats have all bonds in their carbon chains filled or saturated with hydrogen and are usually solids at room temperature. Animal fats are primarily saturated. It is the consumption of too much of these saturated fats which over a period of years is believed to be the primary cause of cardiovascular or heart disease.

Unsaturated fats have bonds on their carbon chains that are not filled or are unsaturated with hydrogen. These places of unsaturation form double bonds between carbon atoms in their chain. Unsaturated fats are usually liquids called oils at room temperature and are generally derived from vegetable sources such as peanuts, cottonseeds, and soybeans.

Polyunsaturated fats are unsaturated fats having two or more places in the carbon chains that aren't filled with hydrogen. These polyunsaturated fats are required by man, but man cannot make them. Therefore, they must be present in the diet.

Hydrogenated fats or oils are fats that have been subjected to hydrogenation — a process whereby hydrogen is added to the fat, filling its "unsaturated" bonds. Such a process is said to produce a hardened fat because it typically converts an oil partially or completely to a fat or a solid. Fats that are solids at room temperature are called *fats* whereas fats that are liquids at room temperature are called *oils*.

Partially hydrogenated fats have had a portion or part of their unsaturated bonds filled with hydrogen. Since hydrogenation is a gradual process filling more and more unsaturated bonds with hydrogen, it can be stopped at any point so that the oil's hardness (or melting point) can be made to order.

Due to the high cost or inaccessibility of butter during World War II, hardened vegetable oils or margarines began to be used as spreads. Although the hydrogenation process converts an expensive oil to a marketable margarine, it also destroys, at least partially, its nutritional value, by converting the essential polyunsaturated fat to a *non-essential* saturated fat. Since the proportion of these two fats is critical to a fat's nutritional value, one day the process of hydrogenation will be regulated or controlled in such a way as to make the most nutritious yet marketable margarine. Another way of improving a fat's nutritional value is to shorten the chain length or select oils that have the desirable chain length.

The majority of the edible oils in this country are obtained from corn, cottonseed, soybeans, olives, and peanuts. They are used in a wide variety of food products ranging from cooking oils to margarines. Several margarine manufacturers have prepared products for partial hydrogenation that are supposed to have all the characteristics of margarine, yet contain significant quantities of unaltered vegetable oils.

Question: **Many athletes avoid eating breads and cereals. How important are breads and cereals in supplying nutrients?**

Answer: Enriched cereal foods, which include bread, cereal, flour, and macaroni products, are important for athletes' body growth and repair. Whole grain and enriched cereal products offer a readily available and inexpensive supply of important amounts of protein, thiamine, riboflavin, niacin, and iron as well as other vitamins and minerals. They are also excellent sources of energy. As a source of thiamine, cereal products are especially important because there are only a few other foods that contain appreciable amounts of this vitamin. The protein in bread and cereals joins those in milk and meat products to help in building body tissues, while iron provided by cereals is an important component of hemoglobin in red blood cells.

Read labels on bread, flour, and other cereal products to be sure that you get the most food value for the money spent. When applied to cereal products: (1) "Enriched" means that extra amounts of thiamine, niacin, riboflavin, and iron have been added by either the miller or baker during the processing of the product; and (2) "Restored" means that products, such as breakfast cereals that have lost food value during manufacturing, have been restored to their original food value during the remainder of the processing. Make sure the cereal products that you purchase are labeled whole grain, enriched, or restored.

Question: **Are coffee, tea, and cola beverages harmful to athletes because of their caffeine content?**

Answer: Tolerance to caffeine varies widely among individuals. A normal person can tolerate the amount of caffeine in most beverages without apparent discomfort. However, people with such illnesses as active peptic ulcer, hypertension, and cardiovascular as well as nervous disorders usually must restrict their intake of products containing caffeine because of the stimulating effect. There is no evidence to show that small amounts of these beverages are harmful in a training diet. On the other hand, there is a good reason for the athlete to avoid them just before an event. Coffee, tea, and cola, while stimulants, may have a depressing effect on the athletes three or four hours later and possibly impair performane if consumed at the meal preceding exercise.

A five ounce cup of coffee, prepared from 15 to 17 grams of coffee, contains about 18 mg. of caffeine per fluid ounce or a total of 90 mg. The caffeine of coffee, among other effects on the nervous system, may cause sleeplessness in some people. A cup of tea contains approximately 12 to 15 mg. of a related stimulant per fluid ounce or 60 to 75 mg. per cup. Cola drinks contain caffeine in amounts ranging from 18 to 28 mg. for a 6 ounce bottle of cola.

Question: **Many coaches advise athletes to avoid "irritating" foods such as spices and "bulky" foods such as lettuce and bran. They in turn recommend "bland and non-irritating" foods. Is there any truth to this advice?**

Answer: The attitudes and ideas that coaches have about which foods are "bland" or "irritating" are usually based on unverified impressions, traditional lore, or their own particular experiences. Reliable studies on this subject fail to substantiate various popular beliefs concerning the effects of food on digestion. The discomfort or difficulties caused by various foods depends most likely on the particular individual. With reference to these foods, modification of eating habits or foods consumed should be based on the athlete's previous experiences.

While black pepper, chili pepper, cloves, and mustard seed may be "irritating" to some, there seems to be no reason for limiting the use of other spices such as paprika, cinnamon, allspice, mace, thyme, and sage. Lettuce, often considered a roughage or bulk type vegetable, actually contains only 1.6 to 4.5 percent of indigestible fiber. Lettuce and other fruits and vegetables of even higher fiber content do not upset the process of digestion. On the contrary, fiber is necessary for normal intestinal function and regularity. However, these foods do increase fecal bulk. Therefore, they are best reduced in the 24 hours preceding the competition or athletic event.

Question: **Is it true that certain foods "burn up" faster than others? Are there various "catabolic" foods that can help you to lose weight?**

Answer: The speed with which food is digested (burned up) or absorbed doesn't affect the caloric value of the diet. Regardless of the time required for digestion and absorption, calories will be converted to fatty tissue if their total intake exceeds energy needs of the body.

There are no foods designated as catabolic. "Catabolic" refers to the process wherein proteins, fats, and carbohydrates are broken down. For example: when extra amounts of these nutrients are consumed; whenever dietary restrictions are imposed and stored materials must be raided for use; to provide energy for cell work; to provide building blocks for synthesis of various tissue components by cells; and to prepare cell wastes for excretion.

Catabolism goes on all the time because cells require energy, building blocks, and must excrete wastes all the time. However, the rate of catabolism increases whenever any of these conditions increases, for example: overeating, increased physical activity (work), rehabilitation from wasting diseases, increased body temperature from fever, or very hot environment.

Knowledge of the satiety value (feeling of satisfaction or fullness) of certain foods may be helpful when trying to achieve weight reduction. Low-calorie diets should be as satisfying as possible. Therefore, foods containing protein and moderate amounts of fat should be included. You should now realize that protein and fat have a "staying power" in the stomach, whereas foods predominantly high in carbohydrate leave the stomach rather quickly.

Question: **What about the consumption of fattening foods such as potatoes, gravy, and candies? Should they be limited in the diet?**

Answer: It is a misnomer to label any food as "fattening." The total caloric intake each day makes the difference, not the presence of one particular food. If you ate 3 cups of mashed potatoes (about 735 calories) every day and excluded all other foods, you would lose weight. Why? Because the total number of calories consumed would be less than the calories expended. There are foods that only supply energy and no other nutrients. These foods should be limited if you are having trouble losing weight and still meeting all your nutrient requirements.

Question: **Is it true that grapefruit has a component which oxidizes or dissolves fat and thus would be beneficial in a reducing diet?**

Answer: There is nothing magic about grapefruit in regard to losing weight. Again, it is a matter of caloric intake and caloric expenditure. Grapefruit is a nutritious low-calorie, high-fiber fruit that tends to satisfy the appetite rather well, as would most other fresh fruits.

Although the processes of mobilization of stored fat and subsequent utilization of it to meet the energy needs of cells is complicated and in part under hormonal control, it really depends on whether the caloric intake is adequate to meet the current energy needs of the body. The body prefers to keep its energy reserve (stored fat) intact and use the energy provided in the diet first.

Fat or energy can't be excreted from your body. As a result something must be done with the extra energy sources you eat and there are only two possibilities: (1) your body can store it in the form of fat, or (2) it can oxidize it if demanded by cell or body need. Fat can only be eliminated from the body after it is oxidized to carbon dioxide and water.

Question: **When young people graduate from high school or college they often tend to gain weight. Why is this so?**

Answer: The typical general pattern of activity for young people in America is toward a decrease whenever they finish their formal education. Opportunities for athletic competition and other physical activities as well as a concern for maintaining one's figure tend to be associated with attendance at school or college. Once a person graduates and/or marries, he usually *decreases* his activity but *maintains* his customary eating habits. Consequently, he overeats and gains weight.

For example, the active girl of 16 or 17 years of age has a daily caloric requirement of about 300 calories more than the same girl at 21 or 22 years of age. Similarly, the young male athlete, active first in high school and then in college sports, may also gain weight,with this increase due both to continuing growth and an increase in muscle mass. The conditioned athlete eating a high-caloric diet will support a minimum amount of body fat as long as he maintains a vigorous program of exercise and activity. However, once he goes out of training, the proportion of his muscle mass will decrease and that of his body fat will increase within a few years. And this undesirable change may not be reflected by a change in body weight, although often it does increase. Consequently, muscle tone, overall vitality, resistance to disease as well as body weight, etc. must all be considered when estimating one's ideal body weight.

The decreased need of calories for growth after adolescence, plus the frequent shift from an active life to a sedentary one, usually produces a tendency to gain weight. From this point of view, all people should count on reducing their caloric intake after graduation, marriage, in their early 20's, or once their total activity is reduced.

Question: **I need to gain at least 20 pounds to make the team. Any suggestions?**

Answer: Gaining weight is one thing, while gaining muscle is totally different. You can gain weight by force feeding yourself, but most of this weight will be fat. There are 3,500 calories in a pound of fat, so all you have to do is eat 1,000 extra calories a day and you'll gain two pounds a week of useless fat!

What you want to do is to gain solid muscle, rather than fat. A pound of muscle contains only 600 calories (and a lot of water), but eating an extra 600 calories a day won't make any difference as far as building muscle is concerned, *unless you've stimulated muscular growth beforehand*. Muscular growth is stimulated best by a program of progressive resistance exercise performed in a high-intensity fashion.

The quickest and best way to exercise is to use the Nautilus machines, which provide full-range exercise. If they are not available in your high school or training center, then select a few good barbell exercises (squat, pullover, press, bench press, curl, deadlift) and perform them three times per week. Properly performed, these exercises should allow you to gain one to two pounds of muscle a week for several months.

Question: **What's the difference between fat and muscle?**
Answer: If we chemically analyzed a pound of fat and a pound of muscle, we'd discover some interesting facts. Both fat and muscle contain water, lipids (fats), and protein, in varying amounts as follows:

	Water	**Lipids**	**Protein**
Muscle	70%	7%	22%
Fat	22%	72%	6%

Don't forget, a pound of fat has 3,500 calories while a pound of muscle contains only 600 calories. Most of muscle is water, whereas fatty tissue is mainly composed of fat.

Question: **What makes a muscle grow?**
Answer: Muscle growth consists of two parts. One, there must be growth stimulation within the body itself at the basic cellular level. After puberty, this is best accomplished by high-intensity exercise. Two, the proper nutrients must be available for the stimulated cells. Providing large amounts of nutrients, in excess of what your body requires, won't do anything to promote growth of muscle fibers. The growth machinery within the cell must first be turned on. Muscle stimulation must always precede nutrition. If you've stimulated muscular growth, by high-intensity exercise, then your muscles will grow on almost any reasonable diet.

Actually, the chemical reactions inside a growing muscle are much more complicated than just exercising and eating. High-intensity muscular contraction results in the formation of a chemical called creatine. The creatine stimulates the muscle to form more myosin, one of the contraction proteins within the muscle fiber. Thus, contraction of the muscle fiber produces creatine, which in turn causes the muscle to form more myosin, which enables it to undergo stronger contractions. This in turn causes the production of more creatine, and around we go again.

Creatine has been identified as the messenger substance that turns on the R.N.A. (Ribonucleic acid) processing line to produce muscle growth. The R.N.A. molecules within a specialized compartment of the cell literally act like an assembly line and hook together various combinations of amino acids, sometimes in combination with complex sugars and fats, to form different compounds that result in the increased size of certain muscle cells. Remember, you must *first* stimulate growth through high-intensity exercise, and *then* provide the proper nutrients.

Question: **What exactly do you mean by high-intensity exercise?**

Answer: For our purpose, high-intensity exercise means the repetitive performance of a resistance movement that is carried to the point of momentary muscular failure. Generally this means that one set of each exercise should be performed in strict style for approximately 10 repetitions. At least 8 repetitions should be performed, and not more than 12. If you can't make 8 then the resistance is too heavy, and if you can perform more than 12 it is too light. The real key to this technique is "pushing" yourself, or being pushed by someone else, to always perform as many strict repetitions as possible. A set is considered finished when it is momentarily impossible to perform another full repetition in good form.

When you can perform 12 repetitions, add a small amount of resistance (usually 5 or 10 pounds) and reduce the repetitions to 8. Try to add an additional repetition each training day. Always add weight when you can perform 12 or more repetitions in good form.

Question: **Tell me more about good form. What is it?**

Answer: Good form means that you perform all your repetitions in a slow, smooth style. No throwing or jerking or sudden movements should be practiced. And special attention should be given to lowering the resistance (eccentric contraction). Research shows that for building muscular size and strength, lowering the resistance is far more important than raising the resistance. For example, if it takes 2-3 seconds to raise a weight, then it should take 4-5 seconds to lower that same weight. All in all, it should take you about one minute to complete a set of 10 repetitions in good form.

5

Are Proteins Power Packed?

NUMEROUS ATHLETES are of the opinion that proteins are power packed. Tom Burleson of the 1972 U.S. Basketball Team and the tallest Olympic competitor at seven feet four inches consumes large amounts of high-protein foods, such as meat and milk, each day. The 1973 indoor record holder in the shotput, Al Feuerbach, in addition to a high-protein diet, regularly takes protein pills. Furthermore, John Smith, world record holder for the 440-yard run recently commented about his diet, "I take a high-protein supplement each day. I figure its better to have too much than not enough."

Some of the reasoning behind massive protein intake by athletes is stated by Chris Fisher of the Australian track team and finalist in the 1500-meter run at the Munich Olympics: "I regularly take protein supplements. When I am training hard and tearing down muscle tissue, I've got to have it in order to recover."

A similar view is adhered to by Russian Olympic champion in weightlifting, Vassili Alexeev. Alexeev tries to consume at least 400 grams of protein a day through massive amounts of foods and supplements.

Among Olympic athletes, there are those who don't believe that high-protein foods and supplements are necessary for maximum performance. These are the thoughts of Nicolo Ciancio of the Australian weightlifting team and the current record holder in the middle heavyweight class: "I was given several weeks supply of protein supplements, but I haven't taken any of them. I don't think they are necessary for strength gains."

In addition, Chris Taylor of the U.S. Wrestling team and the 1972 National Collegiate Champion and heaviest man in the Olympics at 444 pounds noted, "I don't believe in supplements, just a lot of regular food." Steve Genter, silver medal winner in the 200-meter and 400-meter freestyle swimming events, agrees with Taylor as he states, "I take no food supplements as I try to eat a balanced diet each day."

But the dilemma still exists: Are proteins power packed? Should massive protein intake be considered an essential part of the training programs for athletes? And can massive protein intakes be harmful to the body? You will find the answers to these and many more questions within this chapter.

PROTEIN QUALITY

Before you can make specific applications or judgments regarding the value and necessity of following various dietary recommendations concerning proteins, you must become familiar with some background or more basic information about the utilization of protein by the body.

Proteins are very large and complex molecules composed of about 25 different amino acids. They have an average molecular weight of about 36,000 and vary greatly in complexity and structure. Proteins always contain carbon, oxygen, hydrogen, and nitrogen but they may also contain phosphorus, sulfur, iron, and other elements.

Dietary proteins can't be utilized directly by our bodies, as the molecules are too large to pass through the fine pores in the intestinal wall. Therefore, these proteins are broken down almost entirely to amino acids by enzymes in the digestive tract. These small amino acid molecules are able to pass through the walls of the intestine and are then carried by the blood to every cell in the body. Each species and tissue has its own specific kinds of protein that its cells are able to synthesize from the 25 amino acids or building blocks brought to them by the blood following a meal. Proteins are the chief constituents of every cell making up almost half of its solid material (excluding water). In fact, it is the variations of protein in a cell that determine its nature, properties and function. Every living organism depends upon an adequate source of high-quality proteins; they are essential for life.

In order to select adequate sources of dietary protein, it is important that athletes understand the concept of protein quality. Proteins may be classified simply in two categories: high quality or complete proteins and poor quality or incomplete proteins. The high-quality protein has an amino acid composition closer to that of animal tissues and human requirements than a poor-quality protein. Body or tissue proteins are also composed of amino acids, some of which the body cannot synthesize and must therefore be provided in the diet. Consequently, the food that has the greatest amount of these so-called "essential amino acids" present in it has the highest quality or biological value.

The ultimate source of proteins is plants. Animals can't "fix" nitrogen in their tissue like plants can, and therefore, they must obtain their proteins or nitrogenous compounds from plants or other animals that have consumed plants. Proteins from plant and animal tissue aren't of the same quality because they don't contain the same amount or the same kinds of amino acids. It turns out that the food items which supply the highest quality proteins for the athlete come from animal tissues like beef, pork, fish, chicken, eggs, and dairy products. This isn't surprising when you realize that the composition of animal tissues would be more similar to that of human tissues than the composition of plant tissues. In other words, you are more like a cow than a carrot.

IMPORTANCE OF DIETARY PROTEINS

Some nutritionists have said that the most serious nutritional problem in the world today is protein malnutrition. If protein malnutrition isn't the most serious problem, it surely is very close. This is a fact for two reasons: (1) the most costly items in the food budget are those foods containing large amounts of protein; and (2) of these foods, the ones providing the highest quality protein are the most expensive.

It is doubtful, however, that few if any American college athletes suffer from protein malnutrition. Most of these athletes are members of college teams that provide well-stocked training tables. On the other hand, it is quite possible that many teenage athletes, because of their poor eating habits, are not consuming adequate dietary protein.

There are many ways in which high-quality dietary protein can be provided in an athlete's training diet. Animal proteins would provide the necessary amino acids at the tissue site required for tissue protein synthesis. A mixture of vegetable protein could also provide the same amino acids as long as the particular vegetable proteins didn't have the same deficient amino acids. For example, corn protein doesn't have adequate amounts of lysine and tryptophan, which are two essential amino acids for man. However, if it is consumed with beans, which do contain these two amino acids, the mixture would provide a high-quality protein blend. In order to insure that the dietary protein is adequate, you could consume either a one to one mixture of animal and vegetable protein foods or a vegetable protein mixture that doesn't have the same deficient amino acids.

Proteins of excellent nutritive value are readily available in the United States. Figure 5-1 shows the protein content of various foods commonly eaten by American athletes.

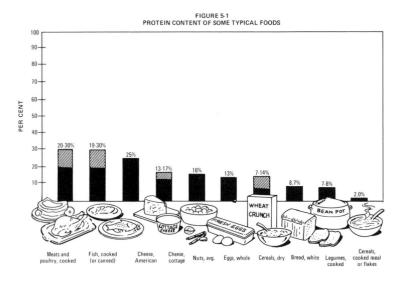

FIGURE 5-1
PROTEIN CONTENT OF SOME TYPICAL FOODS

FUNCTIONS OF PROTEINS

Although the provision of energy is the major and primary function that food performs in your body, any of the major nutrients can be used to satisfy this function, i.e., carbohydrates, fats and, if necessary, proteins. On the other hand, there is no substitute for dietary proteins: the very specific functions they perform in the body are of crucial significance to life.

Proteins are the major organic materials as well as the most important constituents of blood. They are of vital importance (necessary for life) to the structure and function of every cell as well as the means by which cells are interalated to one another.

Proteins are required by your body, in general, for the growth or development of new tissues (especially important for teenage athletes) as well as for the replacement and maintenance of existing tissues. Amino acids are also used in the synthesis of substances essential to body function, such as the enzymes, antibodies, and some of the hormones; and as a source of energy in certain situations.

REQUIREMENT OF DIETARY PROTEINS

The amount of dietary protein required for the functions discussed above has been studied extensively and dietary recommendations have been developed for people of all ages. These are shown graphically in Figure 5-2.

FIGURE 5-2

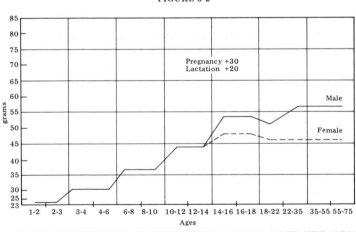

GRAPHIC REPRESENTATION OF RECOMMENDED DIETARY ALLOWANCES (RDA) FOR PROTEIN THROUGHOUT THE LIFE CYCLE (IN GRAMS PER DAY).

The amount of dietary protein, which is actually required for optimum health, is influenced by several factors. Some of these factors relate to the diet while others relate to the individual. In order for an interested athlete to derive the maximum benefit from his dietary proteins, several factors that affect the utilization of proteins must operate.

81

1. Quality of dietary protein. Amount and proportion of:
   A. Essential amino acids
   B. Non-essential amino acids
2. Physiological availability of dietary protein:
   A. Digestion of protein
   B. Absorption of amino acids
3. Adequacy of the diet (non-protein components):
   A. Energy or calorie content
   B. Vitamin content
   C. Mineral content
4. Health of the athlete
5. Frequency of the meals or protein consumption so that all essential amino acids are available most of the time.
6. Rehabilitation from wasting diseases.
7. Physical activity. Prolonged and progressive activity produces a very *slight* increase in protein requirement and an appreciable increase in caloric requirement.

QUESTIONS AND ANSWERS CONCERNING DIETARY PROTEINS AND ATHLETIC PERFORMANCE

Question: **What are protein foods? I'm confused as to the meaning.**

Answer: Protein, itself, is a complex combination of molecules that are made up of amino acids. When we eat a source of protein, chemicals in the stomach act on the protein to liberate the amino acids. Thus protein foods are foods that contain appreciable amounts of amino acids. Meat, dairy products, chicken, and fish are examples of protein foods.

There is also another type of commercially prepared protein food, the increasingly popular protein supplements, which include protein pills and protein powders. They are made from such things as skimmed milk powder, powdered liver, yeast, egg whites, beef organs, calcium caseinate, and soy beans. Most brands carry wording on the label that is similar to "Super-Protein" or "High-Protein," and contain around 90 percent protein with very small amounts of fat and carbohydrate. They are, however, rather expensive at $5.00 or more a pound.

Question: **Advertisers and educators have talked about complete and incomplete proteins, animal and vegetable proteins, and high-quality and low-quality or balanced** and unbalanced proteins. Also the terms "power-packed" and "go-power" proteins are becoming more prevalent. What does it all mean?

Answer: Proteins are composed of amino acids. These simple components are reassembled following digestion to form body tissue, enzymes, and hormones. The nutritional value of a protein depends upon its amino acid composition. Generally, proteins from animal sources are of higher quality or more balanced or complete than those from vegetable sources because the animal proteins contain greater quantities of the amino acids required by man.

The fact that food, when consumed, is generally mixed with other food proteins is often overlooked when a food is promoted on the basis of its quality or quantity of protein. Proteins provided by combinations of cereals and vegetables or combinations of these foods with foods from animal sources, such as cereal and milk, are usually of high value. A varied diet with reasonable food intake contains many different sources of proteins, and the resulting combinations are more than adequate to meet protein requirements. There is no question, however, that an adequate protein intake is essential. Generous quantities are provided in meats, poultry, fish, eggs, nuts, beans, whole grains, cereals, milk, and cheese.

Although proteins can be used as energy sources if necessary, energy is almost always provided by carbohydrates and fats. These two nutrients are much preferred as energy sources, being more easily utilized in the body and much cheaper than protein-rich foods. Therefore, the promotions of "power-packed" or "go-power proteins" is a sales gimmick, which is theoretically valid, but only occurs under such unusual conditions as starvation or an all-meat diet.

Question: **Should massive protein intake be considered an essential part of the training program for athletes?**

Answer: Various reports suggest that many coaches recommend the consumption of large amounts of dietary protein especially for athletes engaged in training. For example, beef steaks are frequently served each day to football players. The Olympic Weightlifting Coach, Bob Hoffman, recommends that athletes consume at least 300 grams of protein a day. Furthermore, many athletes consume various kinds of protein powders and pills, insisting that these are an essential part of their training programs.

No doubt many coaches and athletes reason that the deposition of muscle tissue as well as vigorous activity, which produces an extra "wear and tear" on the body, must produce an increase in the dietary protein requirement. Recently, a leading manufacturer of protein supplements reported that he produces over 100 million protein pills a month.

Although scientists have not always agreed on the amount of protein required by athletes, they have not recommended amounts greater than 150 grams a day. Early German nutrition scientists recommended the consumption of 100 to 150 grams of protein a day. However, around 1900 these recommendations were questioned by Dr. Russell Chittenden of Yale University, who reduced his protein intake and that of his associates to 35 to 45 grams a day for a period of nine months. During this period the subjects maintained their constant body weight while carrying on many strenuous activities. He also noted that the protein content of the body remained constant and that their health and vigor were maintained.

To test his thesis further, Dr. Chittenden studied eight athletes: long-distance runners, the captain of a basketball team, and several gymnasts. These men consumed only 35 to 50 grams of protein a day for six months. All eight of these men competed in athletic contests during this period, and some of them won international championships. These results strongly suggested that athletes who engage in vigorous activities can remain in excellent condition even though they eat much less protein than was recommended by the German scientists or the generous Recommended Dietary Allowances.

Scientists and researchers have repeatedly confirmed the conclusions of Chittenden. There is no scientific evidence available that supports the popular idea that man requires massive amounts of protein-rich food as a result of strenuous activities.

Question: **I'm interested in weightlifting and body building. Since muscular size and strength are important to me, I'll need to consume extra protein. Right?**

Answer: It does seem as though extra protein would be needed for building large muscles, especially since muscles are made up of protein. However, if we look closely at this assumption, we'll see some misleading statements. If you chemically analyzed a muscle from your body, you'd find that over 70 percent of it would be composed of water. Only 22 percent of your muscle is composed of protein.

What does this mean to a weightlifter or bodybuilder? Simply that it takes very little protein to produce a pound of muscle, particularly since so little muscular growth actually takes place within a given 24-hour period. A normal diet will supply you with more than enough protein to build muscles, providing the muscles are first trained in the proper manner.

The results of an investigation by Drs. P. J. Rasch and W. R. Pierson of the California College of Medicine reported in the *American Journal of Clinical Nutrition* (1962) confirm these conclusions. They placed 30 male medical students on a program of progressive resistance exercise (weightlifting). Half of the subjects consumed a commercial protein supplement in tablet form and the other half received placebos (inert, non-protein control tablets), in addition to their normal mixed diets. At the end of six weeks of training and supplementation, there were no significant differences between the two groups with respect to changes in body weight, arm volume, upper arm girth, and strength.

Question: Is all of your knowledge on this subject theoretical or do you have any first hand knowledge that protein supplements are not necessary for muscle building?

Answer: For six years I (Ellington Darden) was a firm believer in high-protein supplements and vitamin pills as well as various other so called "health foods." I took vitamin B_{12} for endurance, wheat germ oil for energy, garlic for purifying the blood, kelp tablets for muscle definition, and vitamin B_6 for strength. At the same time I avoided white bread, carbonated drinks, ice cream, and most carbohydrate foods.

Why did I follow this diet? Mainly because I was convinced that the quickest way to become a physique champion was to follow such a program of eating. Where did I get these beliefs? The majority of them came from the popular weight training and bodybuilding magazines. According to the periodicals, most of the recent contest winners had followed such a program. It was not unusual to read a testimony that such a diet was at least 75 percent responsible for their being a champion.

I never questioned these concepts until I entered graduate school at Florida State University. In fact, most of the time I was trying to find new ways or more concentrated protein supplements to be certain that I was consuming over 300 grams of protein a day.

During my first year at FSU, I attended a graduate seminar at which Dr. Harold E. Schendel gave a two hour lecture on the role of nutrition in physical fitness. Dr. Schendel was professor of nutrition at FSU, but had spent four years previously in Africa and elsewhere directing research on problems of protein malnutrition. He has published over 70 papers in this and related areas.

After our initial meeting, we spent many hours discussing the subject of what effect various foods and eating habits have on athletic performance in general and body building in particular. To say the least, Dr. Schendel disagreed with most of my nutritional concepts and did not believe that my special eating habits or diet were necessary, beneficial, or even safe. His point was that an athlete did *not* require large amounts of vitamins, proteins, or any "health foods." Since I was so convinced about the value of my diet, he didn't argue with me. Rather, he suggested that I read the research literature on this subject and decide for myself what was the best diet for an athlete.

Needless to say, I was not convinced by Dr. Schendel's arguments. After all, his knowledge was all theoretical but I was actually eating a special diet and "knew" about its value. I was a hard training body builder who was constantly trying to increase muscle bulk and strength and I was not about to change my training program because of any university professor or research work done with rats. The muscle building magazines seemed to make sense to me when they promoted the sale of their protein supplements. They argued that if you want to build (or maintain) large amounts of muscle tissue (which everyone knows is largely protein) you must eat a high-protein diet. I was sure that body builders and weightlifters were different from other athletes in this respect and required extra amounts of various nutrients. Therefore, dietary supplementation was more than justified; it was essential!

Rather than spend time arguing this point, however, Dr. Schendel suggested I conduct an experiment on myself. We decided to determine if a athlete in hard training could use the massive amounts of protein I was eating. We agreed that if my body could not use this amount of protein (but broke it down and discarded its end products in the urine) then it surely must not require it.

In order to do this, we kept precise records of my caloric intake (including supplements) and caloric expenditure (including all training) for a two-month period. We varied the protein intake from less than 100 grams a day to more than 380 grams, most of which was obtained from a 90 percent protein powder. All of my urine was collected during the entire period and analyzed for excreted protein end products.

The results of this two-month study were very interesting and thought-provoking. To my surprise, whenever I consumed over approximately 100 grams of protein a day, it was excreted. Furthermore, my body weight remained relatively stationary throughout the entire period. No difference in strength was noted, regardless of the amount of protein consumed. In fact, when I went off the massive protein diet I noticed an additional surge of energy. This may have been due to the fact that several of the body's tissues and organs must work very hard to metabolize excessive amounts of protein and my body was freed from this cost or burden when I stopped eating the protein.

I personally have not supplemented my diet with protein powder or pills since the spring of 1969. Rather, I have consumed a well-balanced diet composed of a variety of foods. I have managed to win or place high in all the physique contests I've entered since then. In fact, in April of 1972, I won the NCAA Mr. America contest.

These facts from my own personal experience have convinced me that the many "health foods," protein, vitamin and mineral supplements available on the market are not being sold or promoted to meet the unique nutritional requirements of athletes, but rather to make a few people very rich.

Question: **Can massive protein intakes (including protein pills and supplements) provide a psychological benefit for some athletes?**

Answer: Any aspect of athletic training, including the way in which the competitor ties his shoes, may have psychological benefit. Whenever an athlete who is approaching maximum performance in his specialty believes that he has a "secret weapon" or edge on his opponent, he will probably be motivated to exert the necessary extra effort and discipline to improve his performance. Drs. Michio Ikai and the late Arthur Steinhaus of George Williams College found that psychological rather than physiological factors often determine the limit of performance and finally become crucial for the athlete who has achieved a high level of skill. The psychological benefit derived from consuming a supplement alleged to have remarkable powers could make the difference in championship competition. But if this is the only contribution that massive protein intakes are making, then such a nutritional program can't be justified considering its cost and possible health hazard. There are other non-toxic means of motivating the athlete.

Question: **Can massive protein intakes be harmful to the body?**

Answer: Studies conducted on rats suggest that excessive amounts of dietary protein may produce damage. Since muscular growth takes place so slowly and isn't dependent on protein intake, massive amounts of dietary protein or protein supplements aren't required (see above) and actually detract from the athlete's maximum performance and physical fitness. Furthermore, the metabolism and excretion of these non-storable protein loads impose serious stress and cause hypertrophy of several very important tissues, especially the liver and kidney.

Question: **Do women athletes require more protein than men athletes?**

Answer: There is no evidence to show that women need more protein per kilogram of body weight than men, except during pregnancy and lactation. It is true that women generally have a higher percentage of body fat than men; thus, theoretically speaking, they would require slightly less protein. Nevertheless, the National Research Council recommends that both men and women should consume 0.8 grams of protein per kilogram of body weight each day.

Question: **Some athletes advocate a diet of meat and a vitamin-mineral preparation. Is this healthy?**

Answer: Although it is possible to exist on a diet of meat and a vitamin-mineral supplement for a period of time, it is surely not recommended. The almost complete abstinence from eating carbohydrates imposes a number of serious hardships on the body:

1. The body requires a small amount of carbohydrate for use as a source of energy for the brain and nervous tissues.

2. A disturbance in the acid-base balance and a tendency

toward acidosis would also occur. The estimated daily need for about 125 grams of carbohydrates would have to be synthesized from the glycerol of fat and from amino acid breakdown.

3. The almost complete absence of roughage would interfere with digestion, absorption, and excretion to some extent.

4. This type of diet would also be dangerous to anyone susceptible to gout or to uric-acid kidney stones, as well as to anyone predisposed to elevated blood fats and cholesterol.

Question: **Some athletes consume large quantities of certain protein foods such as milk, meat, or eggs. Do any of these protein foods offer special virtues to the athlete?**

Answer: Since no single food provides all the essential nutrients, any diet that contains large amounts of a single food will tend to be unbalanced or deficient in one or more nutrients. Therefore, the best diet will always include a wide range or mixture of foods.

Question: **Is beef steak the best source of protein for the athlete?**

Answer: Beef steak is a good source of high-quality protein, but it does provide undesirable saturated fatty acids. Pork and lamb are just as good as sources of protein, but they also contain undesirable saturated fatty acids. Fish and poultry are actually the most desirable nutritionally, if not fried in deep lard. However, any meat or meat equivalent that an athlete enjoys, such as meatballs, pork ribs, fish, chicken, milk or dairy products, and eggs is a good source of high-quality protein.

Question: **Eggs have long been promoted as being nutritious. Recent reports indicate that eggs should be limited in the diet. Is this true? Many athletes consume raw eggs in milk shakes. Is this advisable?**

Answer: An egg can be considered an excellent source of protein, vitamin A, and iron, and a good source of riboflavin and vitamin D. Each egg also contains approximately 350 mg. of cholesterol. According to the American Heart Association, there seems to be a relationship between cholesterol in the diet and heart disease; therefore, they suggest that no more than three eggs be consumed each week.

Although the addition of raw eggs can improve the flavor and nutritional value of a milk shake, this should be avoided because of the possibility of illness from contaminated eggs. Residual Salmonella organism, which causes food poisoning, can remain on the outside of eggs even after washing. Invisible cracks in the shell may permit passage of the disease organism. Nutritionally, raw eggs are less desirable because they contain avidin (neutralized in cooking), which destroys biotin, a B vitamin. The usual methods of cooking eggs assure a safe product.

Question: **How important is it to drink milk? It seems to upset my stomach.**

Answer: All athletes should have some milk or dairy products every day (at least two servings). However, it is true that some people can't tolerate milk as they are allergic to the lactose in it. In fact, recent findings seem to show that up to 75 percent of black athletes have this problem.

If you are allergic to milk, be sure and eat other dairy products in which the lactose has been either removed or altered (converted to lactic acid) through fermentation. For example, yogurt, buttermilk, and some cheeses. You might also try skim milk and powdered milk.

Question: **Is gelatin an acceptable source of protein for the athlete?**

Answer: Gelatin desserts are popular in training diets and pre-game meals. These desserts are good sources of energy because of the sugar they contain and are easily digested. Gelatin isn't a source of high-quality protein because several essential amino acids are missing; however, this doesn't detract from its usefulness in sufficient quantities to supplement a diet adequate in essential amino acids.

Several early studies credited gelatin with increasing muscle power and reducing fatigue primarily because it contained the amino acid, glycine. Later studies revealed that the so-called positive effects of gelatin were due to the physical training effect.

Question: **I've heard that liver is a high-protein food? How often should it be eaten?**

Answer: Liver is one of the best all-around foods for athletes. It is an excellent source of protein, vitamin A, the B vitamins, and iron. For this reason, nutritionists have advised people to eat liver frequently or about once every two weeks.

Many athletes, however, just don't like the flavor of liver. These people can also select an adequately nutritious diet from other foods. For example: (1) poultry, fish, meat, eggs, milk and milk products provide high-quality protein; (2) meats, egg yolks, dried fruits, green leafy vegetables, and enriched and whole grain cereals provide iron; (3) meats, milk, and cereals contribute B vitamins; (4) deep yellow and green vegetables, whole milk, butter, and margarine provide vitamin A. If you enjoy liver and eat it frequently, the assurance of adequate nutrition may be somewhat more certain, but not necessarily more adequate than for the person who makes proper selection from the other nutritious foods available to him.

Question: **Is peanut butter a good source of protein?**

Answer: The composition of peanut butter varies according to the manufacturer. On the average, peanut butter contains about 25 percent protein, 50 percent oil, with the remaining 25 percent composed of carbohydrate, fiber, salt, and water. Although most manufacturers use peanuts of high quality, peanut butter contains a large amount of calories.

A tablespoon of processed peanut butter contains about four grams of protein. To get the same amount of protein that is contained in a three-ounce hamburger patty, it would be necessary to eat about five or six tablespoons of peanut butter. This amount of peanut butter would add to the diet about 500 calories more than a hamburger patty! Such an addition of calories would be undesirable for those athletes needing to control their body weight. However, it could be a useful supplement to those desiring to gain weight. Nevertheless, peanut butter isn't a complete substitute for meat.

Question: **What about soybeans? Are they a good source of protein for athletes?**

Answer: Soybeans were relatively unknown to consumers in the United States a generation ago. Now soybeans have revolutionized American farming and are a major U.S. cash crop. In fact, soybeans ultimately may revolutionize the food industry as well. Whole soybeans contain about 40 percent protein and 20 percent oil. They are now our major source of edible oil. The bean itself, or the defatted press cake, also constitutes a rich source of protein.

Soybeans are very plentiful and hold great promise as a base foodstuff to help feed overwhelming populations. A soybean protein, which is a granular powder, has been available for a number of years and is used as a food supplement in overseas relief programs. Furthermore, a number of soy milk preparations have been developed both here and abroad as a part of a program to increase the protein intake of infants.

Food scientists have developed methods to produce a whole host of imitation meat items from spun filaments of soy protein. The protein filaments simulate the tissue texture of meat. Appropriate flavors and colors are then added. These products are remarkably similar in appearance, taste, and smell to ham, poultry, or beef, with good resemblance in mouth feel and chewing characteristics. With the addition of vitamins and minerals to the meat-like vegetable derivatives, nutritive values compare favorably with the products they are imitating, plus the retail price is lower than the true meat.

Several large food companies are currently producing a complete line of spun protein-derived products. We will certainly hear more about soybean-based products and other oil seed protein in the future.

Question: **I like pizza! Is it all right to eat it fairly often?**

Answer: Pizza prepared properly with meat or sausage, cheese, and tomatoes is a good source of protein and calcium and also contributes its share of iron, vitamin A and C, and the B-complex vitamins to the daily diet. A small pizza with a large vegetable salad and a glass of milk provides a nutritious meal. Likewise, the same thing could be said about a hamburger.

Question: **Some athletes have been encouraged by various articles to eliminate all dairy products from the diet because a hormone in milk is supposed to cause acne. They are also told to avoid chocolate, nuts, and all fried foods. Are these recommendations reasonable?**

Answer: These recommendations are quite unreasonable and may be detrimental to the health and development of children and adolescents. There is no evidence that milk contains a hormone which causes acne. Milk and dairy products make very significant contributions of many nutrients.

Acne is not caused by improper diet. Chocolate doesn't cause acne. Peanuts don't cause acne. Oil-rich foods don't cause acne. According to the American Medical Association's Committee on

Cutaneous Health and Cosmetics, acne is caused primarily by hyperactive oil glands in the skin. The oil glands over-secrete and become plugged, thus producing acne. The hyperactivity of these glands is presumably caused by hormonal imbalance during adolescence, especially in the early processes of maturation.

For treating acne, the AMA has recommended frequent and thorough (but not abrasive) cleaning of the skin with a good quality soap and hot water. Although diet alone will neither clear the skin nor prevent acne, a well-balanced diet is important to skin health. Since nutrient demands are greatest during the growth phase of adolescence, every effort must be made to assure a good supply of calories, proteins, vitamins, and minerals. To deviate from a balanced diet in an attempt to clear up acne is not only foolish, it is very hazardous.

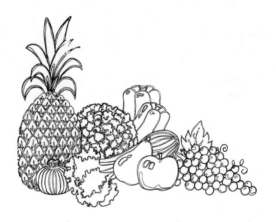

6

Vitamins, Vitamins Everywhere!

THE INGESTION of huge quantities of vitamin pills has become a way of life with some athletes. This is especially true in the United States since we are a "pill-taking" culture. Many of the Olympic competitors in Munich consumed dozens of vitamin pills each day. For example, Phil Grippaldi of the U.S. weightlifting team and several times American champion in the middle heavyweight class had this to say: "I take seven individual vitamin pills at each meal and also several desiccated liver tablets." When asked if he thought they did him any good, he replied, "Well, I've been taking them for so long that I don't want to stop taking them now." Similar practices are adhered to by Deanne Wilson, American champion in the women's high jump: "I take twelve different vitamin and mineral pills every other day — I think they help me."

In addition, Leonard Hilton, National Indoor Champion in the three-mile run recently stated, "I'm a strong believer in additional supplementation. I take vitamin C, E and B complex tablets each day." The bronze medal winner in the high jump at the 1972 Olympics, Dwight Stones, also consumes many vitamins during his training. "I take a multivitamin, plus additional vitamin C and E tablets each day. I think these help me guard against colds and infections."

An interesting joke concerning the athletes from the USA is told by Dr. Daniel Hanley, the chairman of the United States Olympic Medical and Training Services Committee. "Do you know how to tell an American athlete? Answer: He's the one with the most expensive urine in the world. It's full of vitamins." From various observations made at the Munich Olympics, most of the American athletes did consume vitamin supplements each day.

However, on the other side of the coin, there are many Olympic athletes that don't believe vitamin supplements are necessary for optimum performance. Mark Spitz, the American swimmer who won a record seven gold medals, had this to say in an interview: "No, I don't take any food supplements. Some of the swimmers are pill freaks, especially B_6 and B_{12}. I think it gives them just a mental lift — a type of placebo power."

In the same light, John Akii-Bua of the Uganda track team and Olympic champion and world record holder in the 400-meter hurdles commented: "I don't take any supplements. However, I do eat a lot of fresh meat and vegetables." Jim Ryun, the former holder of the world record in the mile agrees in that he consumes no special foods and takes no vitamin supplements in his training. Neither Ryun nor Akii-Bua thinks vitamin supplementation contributes to his physical performance.

Naturally there are many controversial recommendations concerning athletes' use of vitamin supplements. However, before specific questions and answers are presented, it is important that you have a general idea of the functions, requirements, and food sources of the different vitamins. In this respect, you will have a better understanding of the rationale behind the answers to the questions.

Although the early Greek physicians were at least partially aware of the relationship between adequate diets and health, vitamins were not discovered until the latter part of the 19th century. At that time most scientists believed that man required only three groups of nutrients in his diet: proteins, minerals, and energy from carbohydrates or fats. Around 1880, scientists became aware that in addition to these essential nutrients, animals also required something that was present in certain natural foods for maximum health and long life. These compounds were first called "accessory factors" and later vitamins.

Initially, it appeared there was one "accessory factor" or vitamin. It later became apparent, however, that there were many vitamins and that they did not belong to a single group of compounds like carbohydrates, fats, proteins, or minerals. As the vitamins were discovered, they were identified by various

TABLE 6-1
VITAMINS
THE MICRONUTRIENTS

WHAT THEY ARE	WHAT THEY DO FOR YOU	GOOD FOOD SOURCES	RDA
THE FAT-SOLUBLE VITAMINS			
Vitamin A	Not all vitamin A functions are completely understood, but its use is established as an aid to good sight and the maintenance of healthy epithelial membrane. Deficiencies should be prevented by common foods, for you can determine vitamin A presence by food colors.	Deep-yellow foods (carrots, sweet potatoes, apricots, peaches, cantaloupes, butter and fortified margarine, Cheddar cheese) and dark-green vegetables (spinach, mustard greens, Swiss chard).	5,000 IU a day for men, 4,000 IU for women. *Warning:* Daily doses of more than 50,000 IU can be toxic.
Vitamin D	Essential at all ages for calcium homeostasis (primarily responsible for healthy bones and teeth) and for skeletal growth in children and adolescents.	Simple exposure to sunshine may fill required needs. Fish liver oils are a good source. Because of vitamin D scarcity in food, 400 IU of vitamin D has been added to all forms of fluid milk.	400 IU for children, pregnant women and nursing mothers. Probably less for adults unless there is no exposure to sunlight. *Warning:* Amounts in excess of 1,800 IU per day may be hazardous to children. (A quart of fortified milk contains 400 IU of vitamin D. For other foods, check labels.) Children drinking fortified milk as well as fortified-milk flavorings, fruit drinks, cereals and candy can consume too much vitamin D.
Vitamin E (A-tocopherol)	Its *known* function is to prevent the oxidation of certain needed fatty acids. It protects vitamin A from destruction by oxidation. This is the current-rage vitamin; however, there are no known advantages to large intakes of vitamin E except in cases of malabsorption of fat.	Vegetable oils, legumes, nuts, meats, eggs, leafy vegetables, wheat germ and sprouts, whole grains.	Infants: 5 IU. Adults: 15 IU. Evidence of toxic overdose levels is scarce.
Vitamin K	Primarily involved in blood clotting, or coagulation.	Green leafy vegetables, liver, soy oil, egg yolk, cabbage and cauliflower.	None except in therapeutic adult needs to be dictated by a physician. (Single doses of 1 milligram may be given to infants to prevent hemorrhagic disease.)
THE WATER-SOLUBLE VITAMINS			
Thiamine (B₁)	Acts as a co-enzyme in the metabolism of carbohydrates.	Meat (especially pork), fish, poultry, eggs, whole-grain or enriched breads and cereals, dried peas and beans, wheat germ.	Ranges from 0.2 milligram for infants to a high of 1.8 for males.

	Function	Sources	Requirements
	...has as a coenzyme and carrier of hydrogen. Enters into many body-chemistry processes and can be found in almost every tissue of the body.	...milk, cheese, ice cream, liver, fish, poultry and eggs. Enriched and whole-grain breads and cereals.	Ranges from 0.4 milligram for infants to a high of 2 milligrams for nursing mothers.
Niacin (nicotinic acid, nicotinamide)	Acts as a component to two important co-enzymes. Unlike the other water-soluble vitamins, niacin can be stored to some extent in the liver.	Nut butters, meat, liver, fish (especially canned tuna), poultry, milk, enriched or whole-grain breads and cereals.	RDA for niacin is expressed in equivalents because in addition to the niacin in foods, amino acid trytophan can be converted into niacin by the body. Ranges from 5 milligram equivalents for infants to a high of 20 milligrams for adolescents and nursing mothers.
Biotin	Essential for the activity of many enzyme systems.	When other B vitamins are sufficiently present in foods; so is biotin. Also, intestinal bacteria in healthy people manufacture enough to supply requirements.	None.
Choline	Part of several compounds necessary in certain aspects of nerve function and fat metabolism.	Egg yolk, beef liver, all meats, whole grains, legumes, vegetables and milk.	None.
Folacin (folic acid, pteroylmonoglutamic acid)	Involved with a number of metabolic processes. Deficiencies usually occur only when there is impaired absorption, metabolic derangements or an excessive demand by tissues of the body.	In a wide variety of foods of animal and vegetable origin, particularly in glandular meat, yeast and green leafy vegetables.	400 micrograms a day for adults.
Pantothenic Acid	Involved in many body processes such as the release of energy from carbohydrates and the metabolism of fatty acids.	Widely distributed in animal tissue, whole-grain cereals and legumes.	None. A daily intake of 5 to 10 milligrams is probably adequate for children and adults.
Vitamin B6	Essential nutrient in more than 30 enzyme reactions.	Since B_6 is not a single substance but a collection of them, it is available from both animal and plant sources. Liver, ham, lima beans and corn are good sources.	Ranges from 0.3 milligram for infants to 2.0 milligrams for adults and 2.5 milligrams for pregnant women and nursing mothers.
Vitamin B12	Essential for the normal functioning of all cells.	Predominantly in foods of animal origin; since it is bound to protein, this vitamin can be a problem for strict vegetarians.	3 micrograms for adults, 4 micrograms for pregnant women and 4 micrograms for nursing mothers.
Vitamin C (ascorbic acid)	This vitamin has multiple functions to do with blood vessels, hemoglobin, iron deposits, wound healing and resistance to infection. (This is where the prevalent theory about prevention or cure of the common cold derives.)	Citrus fruits, strawberries, cantaloupe, tomatoes, green peppers, broccoli, raw greens, cabbage, potatoes. This is the dangerously lacking vitamin for followers of the all-grain diets.	Ranges from 35 milligrams for infants to 45 for adults and 60 for pregnant women and nursing mothers.

Inositol now is not thought to be a vitamin, although it is often sold as a food supplement. Nutritionists believe we make all we need in our bodies; it is also amply available in a balanced diet.

Vitamin P is nonexistent. The substance once thought to be this vitamin is now called a bioflavinoid (found chiefly in the white pulp and connective tissue of citrus fruits). It has no known need.

numbers or letters. These designations have been largely replaced by chemical names as their molecular structures have been elucidated.

VITAMINS AS A GROUP

The nutrients required by man can be classified in the following categories:

Macronutrients — required by the cells in relatively large amounts:

1. Carbohydrates
2. Fats
3. Proteins
4. Water

Micronutrients — required by the cells in relatively minute amounts:

1. Minerals
2. Vitamins

The vitamins belong to the group of micronutrients. They are a group of compounds that are very dissimilar chemically but that have been lumped together in one group. Also, they are considered in smaller subgroups depending on their:

1. Solubility
2. Functions performed in the body ("what they do")
3. General mechanisms of action in the body ("how they do it")

In addition, vitamins can be classified according to whether they're soluble in fat or water. The names that have been accepted are as follows:

Fat Soluble Vitamins	Water Soluble Vitamins
Vitamin A	Ascorbic Acid (Vitamin C)
Vitamin D	B-Complex Vitamins
Vitamin E	Thiamin (Vitamin B_1)
Vitamin K	Riboflavin (Vitamin B_2)
	Pyridoxine (Vitamin B_6)
	Nicotinic Acid
	Pantothenic Acid
	Folic Acid
	Vitamin B_{12}
	Biotin

Vitamins occur widely in many foods and are easily provided in a properly prepared (not overcooked) mixed diet containing fresh fruits and vegetables. Vitamins are essential because they can't be synthesized by the body at a sufficient rate to satisfy the body's needs; therefore, they must be present in the diet.

Although the therapeutic effects of vitamin supplementation are very rapid and dramatic in a vitamin-deficient subject, it does not follow that such improvement will occur if the subject had the same symptoms but was not vitamin deficient or if large doses of the vitamin are consumed. That is, such symptoms as lethargy, apathy, loss of appetitie, excessive fatigue, and dry or scaly skin may be due to a vitamin deficiency or they may be due to other non-dietary causes such as: a subclinical infection, insufficient sleep or rest, worry or some other emotional problems.

All of the fat soluble vitamins can be stored to some extent in the body, primarily in the liver. If too much of these vitamins are consumed, they may accumulate in the body to such an extent that they produce toxic symptoms. Furthermore, the supplementation of certain other non-stored vitamins to the diet can also produce toxic symptoms.

Although vitamins are often said to "provide energy," they actually cannot. However, some of them are necessary as parts of enzyme systems for the release of the energy supplied in the diet by carbohydrates, fats, and proteins.

QUESTIONS AND ANSWERS CONCERNING VITAMINS AND ATHLETIC PERFORMANCE

Question: **Do athletes engaged in rigorous training programs require additional vitamin supplementation?**

Answer: The rationale for athletes consuming large quantities of vitamin pills is apparently based on the assumption that vitamin requirements are increased during exercise, or that it's possible to supercharge the cells of the body by providing them with an excess amount of vitamins. Although Dr. Thomas Cureton, a well-known physiologist at the University of Illinois, has written several nutritional articles promoting the use of vitamin supplements by athletes, his documentation of reasoning is unconvincing. Furthermore, nutrition scientists have been unable to demonstrate the effectiveness of such nutrient supplements. There seems to be no scientific basis for either of the above assumptions. Vitamin requirements aren't increased before or during strenuous exercise, and it's impossible to supercharge the tissue since most vitamins can't be stored, and any excess amount is rapidly excreted. Extra amounts of the several vitamins, which can be stored, are either inactive and of no benefit or are toxic, producing very serious symptoms. A healthy athlete ingesting a well-balanced diet receives adequate amounts of all vitamins. Therefore, the use of various vitamin pills without a specific deficiency represents nothing more than the use of expensive placebos.

Question: **Is there any one vitamin that is particularly important to an athlete in training?**
Answer: All of the 50 or more nutrients work together and they all are important to an athlete. There is no particular vitamin or other single nutrient that is especially important. From these nutrients the body synthesizes an estimated 10,000 different compounds that are essential to health and performance. A lack of any one might result in the underproduction of hundreds of the essential compounds, but at the same time, adding large amounts of any one or two nutrients can upset the others. Therefore, the athlete should consume a well-balanced diet composed of a wide variety of foods.

Question: **Do cold weather and increased exercise often associated with winter activities make greater demands on the body for vitamins? If so, is it advisable to take a multivitamin supplement?**
Answer: The basic needs for nutrients is no different in the winter than during the summer. Depending upon the weight of clothing worn, more energy may be needed to keep your body warm when exposure to the cold is extensive, but the average difference between energy needs in warm and cold climate is not great.

There's no need for the athlete to supplement an adequate diet with vitamins during the winter. It has been claimed that large amounts of vitamin C will help protect against flu and the common cold, but no good medical evidence exists to support this claim. Little evidence exists that exercise or heavy work increases vitamin requirements. However, increased activity does increase your caloric requirements and therefore the requirements for vitamins, thiamin and niacin, which are involved in energy release. The Food and Nutrition Board recommends 0.5 mg. of thiamin and 6.6 mg. equivalent of niacin for

100

each 1,000 calories consumed. However, slightly increased amounts of these vitamins are easily supplied in the typical diet consumed in America.

Question: **Is it harmful to take vitamin A in large quantities, e.g. 200,000 USP units per day?**

Answer: The functions of vitamin A relate primarily to eyes and the visual process, to the maintenance of epithelial membranes, and to growth. In addition, vitamin A has sometimes been called or referred to as the "anti-infection vitamin" since it does aid in providing satisfactory protective covering and in maintaining part of your body's defense mechanism. But this does not mean that large quantities of vitamin A will improve your eyesight or help you guard against infection.

At the levels mentioned, you would be getting 40 times the recommended allowances for this vitamin. There are only a few abnormal situations in which physicians prescribe massive doses of vitamins. Since vitamin A is fat soluble, large amounts of the vitamin can cause serious tissue damage. If you've been using large amounts of vitamin A for some time, you would be wise to consult a physician to determine if there have been any adverse effects.

Question: **How much vitamin D must be consumed each day? What are the best sources for this vitamin? Is it possible to obtain too much vitamin D?**

Answer: The major function which vitamin D plays in your body concerns the growth and development of bones and teeth. Consequently, the need for vitamin D is particularly critical during infancy, childhood, pregnancy, and lactation. Vitamin D assists primarily in the absorption of calcium from the intestinal tract into the bloodstream.

The recommended intake of vitamin D for infants and children is 400 USP units per day. This amount of vitamin D will provide for the needs of all infants and children except a very small minority who, because of genetic abnormality, require massive amounts. There is no dietary requirement for vitamin D by adults. A sufficient amount of vitamin precursors are synthesized in the body and converted to the active form in the skin by ultraviolet light when the subject spends a few minutes each day in direct sunlight. A dietary intake of 400 USP units, regardless of sunlight exposure, is generous and entirely adequate. There is, in fact, danger in consuming large amounts of this vitamin since it accumulates in the body and eventually causes toxic symptoms.

Vitamin D is found in very moderate amounts in a few foods such as eggs, some salt water fish, and summer milk. Because this vitamin does not occur commonly in nature, it has been standard practice to fortify milk with 400 units of vitamin D per quart. Fluid whole milk, skim milk, and evaporated milk all have added vitamin D. Most commercial infant formulas are also fortified with vitamin D.

There has been a trend in recent years for some food manufacturers to add vitamin D, along with other vitamins, to various processed foods. However, the Council on Food and Nutrition of the American Medical Association recommends the fortification of milk and margarine with vitamin D and sees no justification for adding this nutrient to other foods such as breakfast cereals, fruit drinks, or candy. Such an addition of vitamins by the manufacturer is done to sell his products and not to correct a nutritional problem in the safest or best way. The American Academy of Pediatrics estimates that it wouldn't be unusual for a child to consume as much as 2,000 USP units of vitamin D per day from vitamin fortified foods and supplements. This amounts to over five times the recommended dietary allowance. A daily intake of 1,800 USP units over prolonged periods of time has been shown to be hazardous to some people.

The tolerance of vitamin D varies with the individual, depending on his endocrine (hormonal) system, exposure to ultraviolet light, and his dietary intake of calcium. Under certain very unusual conditions, a few individuals require massive doses of vitamin D to remain healthy. Such people develop rickets and severe bone deformities or have come under the care of a physician.

Question: **Does wheat germ oil (which contains vitamin E) have a beneficial effect on athletic performance, especially endurance-type activities?**

Answer: Probably more controversy prevails concerning the effects of wheat germ oil and vitamin E on athletic performance than any other supplement. Although wheat germ oil is known to be a potent source of vitamin E and the polyunsaturated fatty acids, the evidence for its value as a nutritional supplement for athletes appears unfounded. Once again, Cureton, who is a physiologist, has described several nutritional experiments he has conducted in the *American Journal of Physiology* (1954), which suggest that wheat germ oil has beneficial effects on the performance of some human subjects in training. However, other investigators haven't been able to confirm the work of Cureton. A medical team headed by Dr. I.M. Sharman of London found that adolescents receiving wheat germ oil capsules did not differ in performance measures from those of a control group who consumed placebos. Similar findings using college students have recently been reported by John W. Siemann and Dr. Ronald Byrd of Florida State University in a 1971 edition of the *Florida Journal of Health, Physical Education and Recreation.*

The importance of vitamin E in the human body appears to lie largely in the fact that it is an antioxidant, which in some ways affects the oxidation-reduction reactions in the body. Because of this, many athletes in intensive training assume that supplemental vitamin E will lead to improved performance, especially in those events requiring a great deal of endurance. Apparently, the occasional beneficial effect of wheat germ oil on the performance of some athletes is of a psychological nature.

Question: **Is vitamin E required by athletes? What foods are good sources of this vitamin?**

Answer: Although vitamin E does not have unusual or unique significance for athletic performance, athletes do require a small amount of vitamin E in their diets. Good sources for this vitamin are green leafy vegetables, whole grain cereals, legumes and nuts. Smaller amounts of vitamin E are found in eggs and meat.

Question: **Much has been written about vitamin C and its importance in preventing the common cold. Since a cold can limit performance, should the athlete consume large doses of vitamin C in order to prevent colds?**

Answer: There is some controversy among medical authorities concerning the use of vitamin C in preventing colds. Most of this controversy involves the recommendations of the chemist Dr. Linus Pauling in his book, *Vitamin C and the Common Cold* (1970). Pauling recommends the ingestion of from 1,000 mg. to 5,000 mg. of vitamin C per day. This is many times over the 45 mg. per day recommended by the National Research Council.

According to *The Miami Herald* (September 3, 1971), most of the nutrition experts that were surveyed were doubtful or critical of Dr. Pauling's conclusions. They noted the fact that some people have adverse reactions to massive doses of vitamin C such as diarrhea and the excretion of extraordinary amounts of urine. Dr. Charles Glen King, who originally isolated vitamin C, reports that excessive amounts of this vitamin increase the risk of kidney and bladder stones. Furthermore, there is evidence in the Russian scientific literature that even smaller amounts than those recommended by Pauling are toxic, causing abortion in pregnant women. While some of Dr. Pauling's claims seem to be justified, more well-controlled and large-scale experiments are needed to answer this important question. To date, excessive amounts of vitamin C have not been shown to prevent respiratory infections or colds.

Vitamin C does play several important roles in the body. It is involved in the formation and maintenance of bones, peridontal tissues, and teeth. In addition, vitamin C deals in wound healing, iron deposits, and the synthesis of adrenal hormones and blood cells. But until more conclusive evidence is available concerning vitamin C and the common cold, the athlete need not consume more vitamin C than the recommended dietary allowance, which can easily be obtained by eating four or more servings of fruits and vegetables or one small glass of fresh or reconstituted orange juice per day.

Question: **What is the relationship between vitamin C requirements and cigarette smoking?**

Answer: At least three recent studies have reported that the blood concentration of vitamin C is lower in smokers than in non-smokers. Smokers were found to retain more vitamin C, when large doses were given, than non-smokers. Retention of a high proportion of the test dose suggests abnormally low-tissue stores of the vitamin. A study of guinea pigs who were exposed to tobacco smoke also revealed that the vitamin C content of the adrenal glands was abnormally reduced. The growth of the guinea pigs also was poorer than that of another group who had not been exposed to smoke. Even more serious, however, is the effect that smoking has on pulmonary function, so important to the performance of all body cells and most athletic events. The instant you inhale cigarette smoke, things begin to happen to your heart, lungs, and body. It starts your heart pounding an extra 15 to 25 beats per minute and raises your blood pressure by 10 to 20 millimeters. In your lungs, smoke chokes the airways and attacks the air sacs, leaving a residue of cancer-causing chemicals. It deposits these and other dangerous poisons in your stomach, kidneys, and bladder. And remember — all this happens with every cigarette you smoke. No smoker is immune.

A teenage athlete who smokes may feel winded under mild stress, even if he smokes only five or six cigarettes a day. The smoker will find himself out of breath more quickly than his non-smoking competitors. Plus, there's always the relationship between smoking and heart disease, lung cancer, and respiratory infections. Don't let smoking keep you from giving your best performance.

Question: **What is vitamin P?**

Answer: In the late 1930's a material was isolated from the peels of citrus fruits and was referred to as "citrin" or vitamin P. Certain therapeutic qualities were attributed to this substance. However, no significant therapeutic effects of this vitamin have been discovered or confirmed. To date, there's no evidence that this nutrient is required by man. In 1950, the Joint Committee on Biochemical Nomenclature of the American Society of Biochemists and the American Institution of Nutrition recommended that the term "vitamin P" no longer be used. In some literature it's still possible that the term "vitamin P" is being used.

During the first half of this century, various materials were found to be present in foods which were shown to be necessary for the growth and general health of rats and other experimental animals. Researchers referred to these growth factors with different names, letters and numbers. Most of these materials were later called vitamins and, once their chemical identity was known were given names. However, several of them are still referred to by letter or number, such as vitamins A, C, D, E, K, B_1, and B_{12}.

Question: **Can athletes obtain more vitamins from raw or cooked vegetables?**

Answer: The answer to this question depends on the vegetables and the cooking procedures. Vitamin C, found in tomatoes is water-soluble and heat-labile so cooking washes some of it out and destroys some of it. Therefore, more vitamin C is obtained in raw tomatoes than cooked tomatoes. On the other hand, vitamin A is fat-soluble and locked inside the cell walls of vegetables. Cooking does a better job of breaking down the cell walls than does chewing. Thus, a cup of diced carrots cooked in the correct way provides more than three times the vitamin A of a cup of raw carrots. Therefore it is recommended that several raw and several cooked vegetables be consumed each day.

Question: **Many athletes take B-complex and vitamin B_{12} injections in hopes of increasing their strength and energy. Is there any scientific justification for this?**

Answer: It is often said that vitamins provide pep or energy and that if you feel listless you should take vitamin supplements. While there are other reasons for feeling listless that are usually more likely and while vitamins aren't a source of fuel, they do permit the release of energy provided by carbohydrates and fats. The vitamins, which are involved primarily in the release of energy, are three members of the B-complex: thiamin (vitamin B_1), riboflavin (vitamin B_2),and niacin. These vitamins perform this function by being incorporated as essential parts of cellular enzymes. Enzymes, which act as the body's catalysts, are made by all cells providing they have been supplied with these vitamins and the essential amino acids.

Since these vitamins are necessary for the release of energy in the body, fresh fruits and vegetables must be part of the athlete's daily diet. But injections of vitamin B_{12} and the B-complex would be beneficial only if the athlete suffers from vitamin deficiencies, has been sick, or is in a run-down condition. These injections may help the athlete to make a rapid recovery. However, for a healthy athlete to take B-complex or vitamin B_{12} injections is merely a waste of money. The excess vitamins would merely be excreted in the urine.

Question: **Are fresh vegetables nutritionally superior to frozen or canned vegetables?**

Answer: The scientific methods used in commercially preserving foods are a guarantee that processed vegetables, whether canned or frozen, will be safe and wholesome.

In the industrial canning process, the vegetable is harvested at the proper time to assure optimal size, appearance, and nutritional value. The product is cooled immediately after picking and rushed to the factory. Once at the factory it is washed and blanched and immediately processed by a short-term, high-temperature process. This cooking process, followed by a very rapid cooling period, is the key to the superiority of industrial procedures over many home procedures. The vegetable is cooled in a closed system with a minimum amount of air and cooking time. Therefore, when you open the can at home, it is necessary only to warm the food prior to serving.

In the freezing process, if vegetables are picked and then quick frozen, the nutrient values are equal to or perhaps even higher than those of fresh vegetables. Many times fresh vegetables have not been properly handled in the chain of farm to market to consumer.

Home grown, freshly harvested vegetables cooked immediately generally won't have greater nutritional value than good quality processed vegetables. Slow-cooking methods used frequently by homemakers often destroy more vitamins than are lost during the industrial canning process. Conversely, fresh vegetables that have been poorly stored at the market may be less nutritious than those freshly picked from a home garden. Fresh vegetables that are locally grown in season are frequently cheaper than the commercially processed vegetables. But sometimes, even in season, fresh vegetables can be more expensive than canned or frozen ones.

Even though there may be significant loss of nutritive value from vegetables during both industrial and home processing, this loss is more significant to the vegetables than to you. Don't be fooled by reports of 10 percent to 20 percent nutrient loss unless you know the amount that remains. Such losses are of little practical significance for anyone who consumes a well-balanced or mixed diet that has not been over-cooked and contains some fresh fruits and vegetables each day.

Question: **If all fruits and vegetables are good for athletes, why then are dark green and deep yellow vegetables stressed so much?**

Answer: Fruits and vegetables that contain similar quantities of nutrients are often combined into general groups in discussing a balanced diet. The dark green and deep yellow vegetables supply important quantities of vitamin A, which is not present in significant quantities in all fruits and vegetables. Furthermore, many of the dark green vegetables can be counted on to provide vitamin C as well as appreciable amounts of iron, riboflavin, calcium, and magnesium.

In this respect, nutritionists wishing to emphasize the importance of vegetable sources of vitamin A recommend that a dark green or deep yellow vegetable be eaten at least every other day. Examples of dark green vegetables are spinach, broccoli, kale, collards, and turnip greens. Deep yellow vegetables are carrots, sweet potatoes, squash, and pumpkin.

Certain vegetables and numerous fruits, particularly citrus fruits, are excellent sources of vitamin C. They should be consumed every day to assure an adequate intake of this vitamin. Examples are oranges, grapefruit, cantaloupe, strawberries, and broccoli. However, the singling out of certain fruits or vegetables should not be interpreted to mean that others are not important. It simply means that such foods are very rich sources of certain nutrients.

Question: **What is meant by whole grained, restored, and enriched when referring to cereals? Are whole-grain products superior in nutritive value to enriched products?**

Answer: A whole-grained cereal is one that contains the three principal parts of the cereal — the inner germ, the endosperm, and the other bran layer. Whole wheat and oats are examples of whole-grained cereals. Enriched or restored cereals are cereal products to which the major nutrients lost during the milling process have been added. Nutrients which most states require to be added back, usually to cereal products, include thiamine, riboflavin, niacin, and iron. Because the process of enrichment returns the important nutrients to the product, there is no great difference between the nutrient value of whole-grain and enriched products.

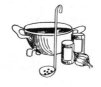

7

Please Pass the Minerals!

VITAMINS HAVE received so much publicity in recent years that it is easy to forget about the need for minerals. Mineral elements originate in the soil and plants grown in the soil take up the inorganic elements they need for forming their roots, stems, and leaves. Animals in turn eat the plants and utilize the minerals they require for their own body development and functioning. Thus, humans obtain mineral elements by eating not only plants but also animal tissue and animal products. Indirectly, the minerals of the soil become the minerals of the body.

FUNCTIONS OF MINERALS

Most of the functions that minerals perform in the body may be listed under three main categories: structural, functional, and regulatory components.

As structural components, minerals provide rigidity and strength to bones and teeth.

As functional components, minerals occur in soft tissues and fluids throughout the body enabling cells to perform many of the functions assigned to them:

1.   They help to maintain the correct total amount of body fluid as well as its distribution throughout the body.
2.   They contribute to the maintenance of a neutral acid-base condition of the blood and body tissues.
3.   They make possible normal rhythm of the heart beat and contractability of all muscles.

4. They help to maintain a normal response of nerves to stimuli.
5. They are essential for blood clot formation.

As regulatory components, minerals occur as essential parts of many enzymes and hormones that regulate or control most of the body's reactions:

1. Iodine —thyroxine
2. Zinc — insulin
3. Sulfur — vitamin B_1
     vitamin biotin
4. Cobalt — vitamin B_{12}
5. Magnesium — enzymes for energy release

While the minerals are identified separately, it should be understood that they act together and in various combinations. Therefore, while certain minerals serve specific purposes in the body, they rarely act alone in accomplishing these purposes.

MINERALS AS A GROUP

The minerals in the body can be separated into two groups: those that occur in the body and in foods in relatively large amounts and those that occur and are needed in minute amounts. The minerals that occur in large amounts are calcium, phosphorus, magnesium, potassium, sodium chloride, and sulfur. The minute or trace elements are composed of iron, copper, iodine, fluoride, cobalt, manganese, and zinc. The National Research Council has established recommended dietary allowances for calcium, phosphorus, magnesium, iron, iodine, and zinc (see Table 7-1). It is believed that if the requirements for these and other nutrients on the recommended dietary allowance table are met, then the remaining minerals will also be present in adequate amounts. Only five minerals will be individually discussed: calcium, phosphorus, magnesium, iron, and iodine.

CALCIUM

Calcium is present in your body to a greater extent than any other mineral. It accounts for about two percent of the body weight of an adult. The largest part of this calcium is in the bones and teeth with very small amounts contained in the soft tissues, blood, and other body fluids. Although the amount of

110

calcium in the soft tissues is small compared with that in the bones, its presence is essential and its concentration must be kept within very narrow limits for the body to function normally. For example, when too little calcium is present, an individual develops, among other symptoms, tetany or violent muscle spasms. On the other hand, when too much is present, calcium may be deposited in the muscles and organs and impair their function.

There are foods available that are excellent sources of calcium. Milk and dairy products are by far the most important foods that contain calcium. Leafy-green vegetables are also good sources of calcium.

PHOSPHORUS

Phosphorus is an important substance in every body tissue. The amount of phosphorus present in the body makes up about one percent of the body weight and is therefore the second most abundant mineral in man. It occurs mainly in combination with calcium in the bones and teeth, but smaller amounts occur in the fluids and soft tissues as parts of any compounds that are necessary for cell function. The phosphorus compounds play an essential role in the release of energy from food and the utilization of that energy by the cell for all its activities.

Most plant and animal foods contain appreciable amounts of phosphorus. Because of the wide distribution of phosphorus in foods, humans are seldom if ever deficient in this mineral. Meat, poultry, fish, eggs, and dried beans are excellent sources of phosphorus.

MAGNESIUM

Magnesium is closely allied to calcium and phosphorus in distribution and function. It is most heavily concentrated in your skeleton with smaller amounts found in your soft tissues and extracellular fluids. The primary function of magnesium appears to be as an activator of certain enzymes in the body, particularly those related to carbohydrate metabolism. Deficiencies of magnesium are rare under normal circumstances, especially if the diet contains a reasonable amount of green vegetables. Magnesium is present in all green plants and nuts.

IRON

Iron is widely distributed in the body in small amounts. Your body normally contains about one-seventh of an ounce of iron, or

TABLE 7-1
MINERALS

WHAT THEY ARE	WHAT THEY DO FOR YOU	GOOD FOOD SOURCES	RDA*
MINERALS.			
Calcium	A major constituent of the body for bones and teeth. A small percentage of it is utilized for control of nerve functions.	Milk, cheese and green leafy vegetables. Without a daily intake of 2 or more glasses of milk or 2 or more servings of cheese, adequate calcium is difficult to get.	800 milligrams for adults.
Phosphorous	Along with calcium, the major constituent of bones and teeth.	Available in major calcium sources, also in meats and cereals. Adequate amounts are easy to get.	800 milligrams for adults.
Copper	An essential for all mammals. Deficiencies in human beings are rare.	Ordinary diets provide 2 to 5 milligrams per day.	2 milligrams for adults.
Fluoride	Incorporated in the structure of bones and teeth and necessary to the resistance of tooth decay.	Fish, cheese, milk are good sources, though not enough to prevent tooth decay. Water supplies that have been treated to bring the fluoride concentration to 1 part per million are.	None, but water fluoridation is recommended where fluoride level is low.
Iodine	Important to the healthy functioning of the thyroid gland. Iodine deficiency may cause goiter.	Seafoods. Use of iodized table salt will preclude deficiency.	Ranges from 35 micrograms for infants to 150 for adolescent males.
Iron	A constituent of hemoglobin and a variety of enzymes. Now considered most lacking nutrient, especially among women.	Red meats, whole grains, wheat germ, prunes, raisins, molasses and dark-green vegetables.	10 milligrams for males. 18 milligrams for females over 10 years of age.
Magnesium	An important constituent of all soft tissue and bone and an activator of many enzymes.	Deficiency in a balanced diet is unlikely.	350 milligrams for men. 300 milligrams for women.
Sodium, Potassium and Chloride	These minerals are often called electrolytes. They maintain an inner balance of body fluids and contribute to cellular enzyme function.	All are readily available in common foods. In fact, sodium (table salt) intake can be harmfully high.	None.
Zinc	Important in taste and smell acuity and wound healing.	Green leafy vegetables, whole grains, and meats.	15 milligrams for adults.
THE TRACE MINERALS			
Chromium, Cobalt, Manganese, Molybdenum, Selenium, and possibly others.	In minute amounts these minerals serve essential body needs.	Green leafy vegetables, whole grains, organ meats and lean meats.	None
Water	Water is not usually counted as a nutrient, but it is well-known that we can survive without food much longer than we can without water.	Water or other fluids.	None, but 1 to 2 quarts of fluid daily is recommended.

Of all the known minerals the body needs, widespread deficiencies exist only in calcium and iron. In some geographic areas, iodine and fluoride supplies are low.

*Recommended Daily Dietary Allowances.

approximately one three-hundredths as much as calcium. The major portion of iron in the body is in the blood, chiefly in the red blood cells as hemoglobin, while the rest is in storage forms. Iron is essential in the formation of hemoglobin molecules, which perform the important operation of carrying oxygen from the lungs to all of the cells in the body. Iron deficiency results in an anemic condition whereby the individual becomes weak, listless, pallid in appearance, and has frequent headaches. This anemia occurs most frequently among infants, young children, and women. In women this condition may occur as a result of large menstrual losses or the increased requirement of pregnancy, which in turn can also produce a deficiency in the newborn infant.

About two-thirds of the iron available to consumers in the United States come from meat, poultry, fish, and enriched flour and cereal products. The most concentrated sources are liver, muscle meats, dried beans, and spinach.

IODINE

Iodine is an essential substance of the hormone thyroxine, which is synthesized by the thyroid gland. Thyroxine plays a vital role in energy metabolism, growth, and mental development of the young, and normal reproduction. Iodine deficiencies may cause both physical and mental retardation in children. An enlargement of the thyroid gland, called goiter, is also a result of iodine deficiency.

Iodine is present in foods in very small amounts and likewise there is only a minute quantity of iodine in the body. Salt-water fish provide rich sources of iodine, but iodized salt is the most dependable source of this mineral for most people.

MINERAL REQUIREMENTS

Recommended dietary allowances for minerals have been established by the National Research Council. Again these recommendations vary according to age, weight, and sex (see Table 7-1).

WATER

Water is an essential nutrient even though it is often neglected when the nutritional needs of the body are discussed. The body's need for water is exceeded only by that for oxygen. The length of time you can do without water depends on the environment. In the middle of the desert on a hot day, you might remain alive for less than 10 hours, while you might remain alive for several days in a more favorable environment. On the other hand, individuals have gone without food for long periods of time and survived, provided they had access to adequate amounts of water.

Approximately 65 percent of your body weight is composed of water. The total water volume is related to the mass of lean tissues of the body rather than to body weight, as fat tissue contains less water than lean tissue. Two-thirds of the body's water is contained within the cells and the remaining one-third is found in spaces outside the cell. Somewhere between three to four quarts of water as blood are constantly circulated to every cell in the body.

FUNCTIONS OF WATER

Water functions in your body as a building material, solvent, lubricant, and temperature regulator. It serves as a building material in the construction of every cell and the different cells vary in their water content. For example, the water content of the following tissues is: teeth — less than 10 percent; bone — 25 percent; striated muscle — 70 percent water.

As a solvent, water is used in the digestive processes where it aids the chewing and softening of food. It also supplies fluid for the digestive juices and facilitates the movement of the food mass along the digestive tract. After digestion, water as blood is the means by which the nutrients are carried to the cells and waste products removed.

Water also serves as a lubricant in the joints and between internal organs. As a lubricant it keeps your body cells moist and permits the passage of substances between the cells and blood vessels. Water also plays the very important function of removing heat from the body as sweat or by its evaporation.

SOURCES OF WATER FOR THE BODY

Water for the body comes from several sources: beverages and liquids of the diet, water contained in the solid foods of the diet,

114

and water produced by the metabolism of the energy nutrients within the tissues. Naturally the largest amount of body water comes from ingested beverages such as water, coffee, tea, milk, and fruit juices. Many solid foods in the diet contain over 70 percent water. Figure 7-2 indicates the percentage of water in some common foods.

FIGURE 7-2

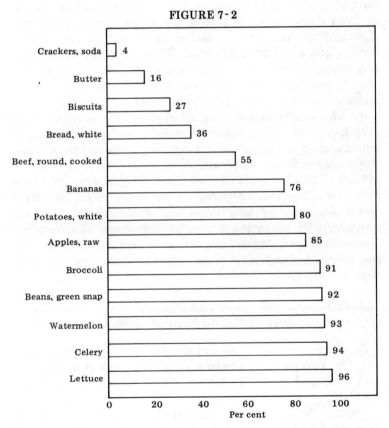

PERCENTAGE OF WATER IN SOME COMMONLY USED FOODS

Water is produced as a by-product whenever carbohydrates, fats, and proteins are utilized in the body. The amount of water produced by different food substances varies according to the

115

following estimated scales:

1 gram of carbohydrate = 0.6 grams of water
1 gram of fat = 1.07 grams of water
1 gram of protein = 0.41 grams of water

REQUIREMENTS FOR WATER

For the young adult and athlete, activity and environmental conditions are the two most important factors that determine the body's need for water. During study, rest, and sleep, the loss of water from your body is small as compared to active exercise such as tennis, soccer, and football. When the temperature is hot and humidity low, more water evaporates from the body surface. In most individuals, thirst or the desire for water is adequate to meet the needs of the body. However, in certain situations where extreme sweating takes place, or where the air is very dry, the thirst mechanism may not allow for the drinking of enough water. In these cases it becomes necessary to increase the intake of fluids. Generally speaking, however, five or six glasses of liquid should be consumed daily by the sedentary individual. Since so many factors affect the requirement for water, there is no single figure that would represent the requirement for all people of a given age or sex. The National Research Council states that a reasonable standard for calculating the daily water allowances is one milliliter per calorie of food.

QUESTIONS AND ANSWERS CONCERNING MINERALS AND ATHLETIC PERFORMANCE

Question: **Are minerals important in preventing severe muscle cramps that sometimes occur in the legs of cyclists, runners, and football players after extreme physical effort?**

Answer: Many factors are involved in the physiological responses of muscles to prolonged exercise, during activity, and during the state of recovery. The tissue content of sodium chloride (table salt) is a critical factor, and this tissue component may be seriously depleted by prolonged physical exercise or perspiration, particularly in hot and humid weather. This depletion has been very prevalent even though the athletes have taken what they believed to be adequate quantities of salt

116

before and during exercise. It was reported in a 1971 edition of the *Journal of the American Medical Association* by Dr. Allan Ryan of the University of Wisconsin, that an athlete may lose as much as three to five grams of salt per liter of sweat. This salt should be replaced by the frequent drinking of salt water (.1 to .2 percent concentrations).

Another factor to be considered in leg cramps is the depletion of glycogen in the muscles. The muscle tissues become strongly acid during vigorous exercise as a result of the accumulation of lactic acid. The normal level for this acid may not be achieved until 24 or more hours after the exercise has been completed. Dr. Ryan, therefore, recommends that muscle cramps might be prevented by giving more attention to adequate consumption of salt water before the event and rapid eating of carbohydrate foods and water following the exercise.

Question: **Is it true that too much calcium in the diet will cause calcium deposits in the joints?**

Answer: Calcium is required in the diet throughout life. Suboptimum calcium intake in adults has been indicated recently as a contributing factor in the development of a disease characterized by weakened bones and invalidism. Optimal calcium nutrition should be promoted for athletes, and one of the best sources of calcium is milk or milk products. The recommended amount of milk for adults is at least one pint per day.

An excessive dietary intake of calcium may cause calcium deposits in the soft tissues of the body, but it will not have any effect on diseases that affect the joints, such as arthritis, gout, and associated conditions. Typically, the protective mechanisms in our body regulate the absorption and output of calcium so that the body retains only a sufficient amount to meet its needs. It should be noted, however, that very excessive intakes of calcium or vitamin D can be detrimental.

A condition known as hypercalcemia, characterized by an excess of calcium in the blood, may develop in certain abnormal individuals or in infants and young children who have consumed an excess of vitamin D. Vitamin D aids in calcium absorption in the body and it appears that excessive amounts of vitamin D can cause an excessive absorption of calcium. This condition can be reversed by decreasing dietary amounts of vitamin D. Hypercalcemia is also found in patients being treated for peptic ulcers with both excessive alkali therapy and

117

excessive milk intake. However, it does not occur in cases where alkali therapy is not used, even if large amounts of milk are consumed.

Question: **If fluoride occurs naturally in foods, why is it necessary to fluoridate public water supplies? What happens to fluoride in the human system?**

Answer: Much attention has been given to the nutrient fluoride over the past several years, especially as it relates to the fluoridation of the public water supply. Fluoride is a very important nutrient and its deficiency has had a serious effect on the health of many Americans. Small amounts of fluoride are present in most foods. Green plants and sea foods are the richest sources, although fluoridated water is the most reliable and certain way of supplying adequate amounts of this nutrient.

Almost all of the body's fluoride (96 percent) is in the bones and teeth where it represents a storage site that can be called on for use elsewhere in the body when the intake is adequate.

Fluoride is involved in the development of strong bones and teeth. It seems to occupy an essential position in the crystalline structure of these tissues and if it is not present in adequate amounts, the bones and teeth are weakened.

The evidence for fluoride deficiency is not very specific. However, it is believed that a major cause of tooth decay and bone disease is the result of fluoride deficiency. The evidence for the relationship of fluoride and tooth decay is overwhelming. It is known that the presence of fluoride in enamel, the crown or exposed part of the tooth, makes it a much harder or stronger tissue. Dental decay has been shown to be reduced over 65 percent among children following the fluoridation of their water supply. Furthermore, there have been fewer missing teeth, less malocclusion (bite contact), and less periodontal (gum) disease. These beneficial effects of fluoridation are most pronounced up to the eighth year of life, but have been shown to be effective through the fourteenth year.

Question: **Do female athletes need special mineral supplements when they compete during their menstrual period?**

Answer: Generally speaking the answer is no. Normal menstruation involves a small loss of iron and protein, and both will easily be replaced by good nutrition throughout the month.

118

However, women with excessive menstrual flow (about five percent of the women) would be wise to increase their consumption of foods which contain iron, especially prior to and during their menstrual period.

Question: **Since so many iron fortified foods are on the market, is there a shortage of iron in the American diet?**

Answer: Iron is an important constituent of blood hemoglobin. Iron reserves in females' bodies are important as a protection against iron depletion when blood is lost during menses and childbirth. Extra iron is also needed during pregnancy and lactation. The amount of dietary iron absorbed from food varies according to need. It is this increased dietary absorption, coupled with adequate body iron reserves, that affords protection against the consequences of iron loss or increased need for iron. A deficiency of iron in the body may express itself in a condition known as anemia, which is characterized by a subnormal amount of iron or hemoglobin in the blood. An anemic person is also weak, listless, has unjustified fatigue, loss of appetite, retarded growth, and reduced resistance to disease. Recent surveys have indicated that most adolescent boys consume a diet containing an adequate amount of iron. However, nutritionists and blood specialists are alarmed by reports that young girls and women consume diets that provide only about half of their iron requirements. In order to meet the needs of this segment of the population, the American Medical Association and the National Research Council recommend a daily intake of at least 18 to 20 milligrams of iron. Studies have found that women, who have a greater need for iron than men, consume on the average only 8 to 10 mg. per day. In this respect, women should be encouraged to eat iron fortified foods as well as iron rich foods such as meat, eggs, green vegetables, and whole-grained and enriched cereals. Furthermore, women who are thinking about starting a family should take steps to build up adequate body stores of iron to see them through their pregnancies.

Adequate fluoride nutrition may be shown to have an even more important effect on bone tissue. One of the most debilitating diseases of older age is the weakening of bone, especially among women.

The skeleton or bone tissue is not static once it is laid down. Rather it represents an emergency source of minerals for use by other cells whenever the diet is inadequate. Since such erosion of bone tissue is very slow and occurs without any immediate clinical effects, it may go on for years unnoticed. Unfortunately, the body cannot replace decayed teeth, and once extensive bone erosion and fractures have occurred, healing is almost non-existent.

Question: **Some people adhere to the notion that the soils of the United States are becoming deficient in minerals, therefore many fruits and vegetables are losing their nutritional value. Is this true?**

Answer: Numerous pseudo-scientists and faddists have long associated the mineral content of the soils too closely with the nutritional status of people living on products of those soils. Various soils do differ in mineral content, but the level of minerals in the vegetation grown from the soils may not reflect those differences. Soil composition doesn't affect plant composition, except for iodine content and possibly fluoride and perhaps the plant's yield, but not nutritive value. Actually the plant's heredity (the kind of seed planted) and the moisture available control the plant's size, shape, and composition.

Question: **Recently, the popular press has made people aware of the use of food additives such as monosodium glutamate and calcium propionate. Why are so many additives used in foods? Is it possible that such additives can be detrimental to athletic performance?**

Answer: Chemical food additives are necessary in preserving the high quality of many foods now available in the supermarket. These chemicals are added by food processors to improve or maintain quality, or to give some added advantage not found in its fresh state but desired by the consumer.

Most consumers are unaware of the vast preparation that goes into many of the foods that are found in today's market. The time involved and distances involved in getting products from farm to manufacturers and then to consumers are sometimes great. It therefore becomes difficult to keep food items at the peak of freshness throughout this entire journey unless food additives are used. Space doesn't permit me to discuss the additives that help to keep foods high in quality until they are ready for use. However, they can be grouped under the heading of nutrient supplements, flavoring agents, preservatives, emulsifiers, and stabilizers and thickeners.

The Food Additives Amendment, passed by the Federal Government in 1958, requires that additives be proven safe for consumption. In this respect a variety of carefully controlled tests are made before additives can be marketed. The athlete need not be worried about certain food additives affecting his performance. These additives are used in such very small amounts that one would have to consume abnormally large amounts of certain foods in order for dangers to even be remotely possible. Most of the additives are completely harmless if consumed in normal amounts.

Question: **If an athlete drinks water during competition, will this be harmful or detrimental to his performance?**

Answer: There are people who think it is harmful to drink water during physical performance. They argue that if an athlete drank all the water he wanted, he would not perform at his maximum. Although this might be true immediately after the intake when the stomach is distended and then as the kidneys deal with the load, or in some very emotional athletes (keyed up athletes could develop stomach cramps from reactions to water), scientific evidence generally does not support any detrimental long-term effect. Excessive water losses through sweat frequently cause mental confusion, which could definitely affect an athlete's performance. More athletes have probably been affected by too little water intake during performance than too much. Therefore, the athlete should generally be allowed to drink as much water as he or she wishes.

Question: **What is the minimum requirement for water per day for an adult?**

Answer: Water is a very important nutrient and an essential component of the body. The body of an adult man contains more than 10 gallons of water! A loss of 10 percent of body weight as water is disabling, and the loss of 15 to 20 percent of body weight as water can be fatal.

The minimum dietary requirement under the most favorable environmental conditions is about one quart of liquid per day for an adult engaged primarily in sedentary activities. This is a true minimum and doesn't provide a margin of safety. A safer recommendation would be a minimum of two quarts per day. Ill health and ultimately death occur if the water requirement is not met. Under ideal conditions, man can survive about 10 days without water although he can go much longer without food.

The requirement for water depends on its loss in the urine, feces, perspiration, and respired air. The loss in the urine is obligatory, since certain waste products can be excreted only by the kidneys with water needed as the solvent. The amount and nature of these waste products and subsequent water requirement depend upon the nature of the diet. For example, the excretion of the end products of protein metabolism requires the most water. Insensible water loss by evaporation from skin and lungs, under the ideal environmental conditions, amounts to about a pint and a half to two pints a day. The amount lost by these routes will vary with the amount of physical activity and climatic or environmental conditions (temperature, humidity, and wind). Water lost by sweating can be enormous, amounting to two or three gallons during a day of hard labor or physical activity in extremely hot weather. Under these conditions, free access to water and frequent replacement of salt loss is vital.

Question: **How much water should an athlete consume during competition?**

Answer: Profuse perspiration is very common for the athlete engaged in rigorous training or competition and may represent a very significant route of loss not only of water, but also sodium, chloride, and potassium. Such a situation can cause rather serious consequences for the athlete intent on performing at his maximum capacity if the water and minerals are not replenished quickly and adequately. The loss of both water and minerals can affect performance by causing muscle cramps, weakness, paralysis, weight loss, and diarrhea. This may result in reduced blood pressure, loss of coordination, impaired respiratory function; and if untreated — death.

Many coaches limit their athletes to small amounts of water during practice or a game. Others use water breaks as a "reward" rather than a necessity. Some allow no water, apparently thinking that this will make the players "tougher" or more disciplined. And there are a few coaches, a very few, who allow their players an unlimited supply of water. Unfortunately, there are no studies available that show how much water an athlete should consume during a contest. Although there is no evidence to support the statement, a current book on sports medicine recommends that an athlete should drink enough water during a game to keep his weight loss to four pounds or less. Since some football players may lose as much as ten pounds during a strenuous practice, this would be quite a lot of water to drink. Small frequent drinks (about two ounces at a time) would seem better suited to meeting these needs than several large amounts. If an athlete is allowed to drink all the water he wants (preferable salt water) during practice or competition, he soon learns what amount best suits his body.

Question: **Athletes tend to sweat profusely when exercising during hot weather. Should salt be taken routinely?**

Answer: Extra salt should only be taken during hot weather under conditions that cause profuse sweating. Copious sweating associated with prolonged and vigorous exercise or hard physical labor in hot weather may cause sufficient sodium loss to produce illness. However, it should be pointed out that the body is able to compensate partially in a few days so that the daily loss of sodium is less as you become accustomed or acclimated.

A biochemistry team in London, headed by Dr. E.M. Clarkson (*British Medical Journal,* September 11, 1971), has recently experimented with a slowly released oral sodium chloride preparation that shows great promise in the future. These tablets are called Slow Sodium and are marketed by Ciba Pharmaceutical Company. English soccer players have successfully used them while competing in hot temperatures. The tablets have been well tolerated with fluids and no players suffered either acute or chronic salt and water depletion. By ingesting a supply of Slow Sodium tablets at a suitable time before an acute sweat loss is about to take place, it is possible for the loss to be at least partially replaced from the gut as it is occurring. With a continuous absorption of salt from the Slow Sodium tablets in the intestine and the frequent drinking of water, the athlete need never suffer from the muscular weakness of excessive sweat loss.

Question: **Much has been said about the athlete who sweats a lot, especially as far as salt replacement is concerned. Is it possible to obtain too much salt?**

Answer: Salt contains about 39 percent sodium. Healthy persons will normally and promptly eliminate the extra amounts of sodium ingested from table salt and from other foods. Persons with kidney dysfunctions may not be able to excrete all of the extra sodium as fast as they should and often retain too much fluid in the body, causing edema. People with a history of circulatory problems such as heart disease, high-blood pressure, and swollen ankles must avoid excessive salt intake since it may aggravate the problem.

Question: **Is there any truth to the common concept of "eat first, drink later?"**

Answer: Whether the liquid is water or another beverage, it is not harmful to drink during a meal. However, it is a bad habit to use excessive amounts of liquid to wash food down without chewing it well. But even then, the digestive juices are usually sufficiently powerful to handle most large pieces of food. Drinking a large volume of beverage just prior to eating could cause distension or give an uncomfortable feeling of fullness and thereby reduce the appetite. Beverages that are cold or iced should be drunk more slowly because if they are consumed quickly, normal stomach functioning may be interrupted. Therefore, common sense should be used by the athlete when it comes to the drinking of liquids with meals.

Question: **What is the value of the action drinks promoted for athletes and other extremely active people?**

Answer: The action drinks include several products new to the beverage market. These products have been referred to as sports drinks, thirst-quenchers, oral electrolyte mixtures, and perhaps other terms. Actually, they are diluted solutions of glucose (a simple sugar), sodium chloride (table salt), and other salts, citric acid, and an artificial sweetener. Although the action drinks were originally prepared for athletes, the manufacturers have broadened their promotions to include all individuals who work hard, play hard, or just get thirsty. And for wider appeal, the beverages now come in several flavors. At least one brand is carbonated and at least one brand has vitamin C added.

These action drinks were designed to serve as thirst-satisfying means of replacing electrolytes (minerals) and water lost in perspiration. One study suggested that the electrolyte solution is much more rapidly absorbed than water. Also, depending on the brand, 200-300 calories may be supplied from sugar in a quart.

The minerals other than sodium found in action drinks are not thought to be of any value. As for sodium, approximately a quart of the beverage must be consumed to supply the equivalent of one gram of salt (or the amount of sodium found in two half-gram salt tablets). When sweating is profuse, large amounts of the electrolyte solutions may serve the same function as salt tablets. If sweating is mild to moderate, the sodium provided by the normal intake of salt in the diet is sufficient.

Concerning athletic performance, there have been no studies that support claims for improved performance resulting from the use of action drinks.

Furthermore, you can make your own action drink, or saline solution, at home for about one tenth the cost. All you need is a quart of water, ½ teaspoon of iodized salt, plus a little sugar and flavoring.

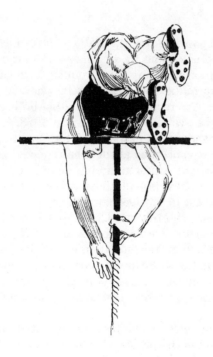

8

Are "Health Foods" Healthful?

PILLS, POTIONS, and powders line the walls of most "health food" stores. These products come in all shapes and sizes and are guaranteed to cure almost anything from the common cold to rheumatism, or to make you a winner in whatever athletic event you compete. As a result, the sales volume of "health food" was estimated to be over a billion dollars in 1973.

In fact, we have moved out of the era of the "health food nut" so that now if you're concerned about "health foods" you are no longer considered a nut! Unfortunately, the uninformed or unscrupulous "experts" have the platform today and have generated fear and distrust in our food supply.

The eminent food scientist and Chancellor Emeritus of the University of California, Emil Mrak, stated in 1970, "Our country has more food and better food than ever before, and more than any country in the world as far as per capita availability is concerned. Furthermore, we have a greater variety and certainly the abundance to enable all of us to be the best fed people in the world."

But we have not selected the best or the nutritionally balanced diet. So what is the problem? Who is to blame? Is it the food industry, the federal Food and Drug Administration, or the American public? Who is exploiting whom? Is it the long time established food industry or the "health food" faddists? What is the real solution to suboptimum health or malnutrition? We seem to know enough; how do we put it into practice now?

126

"Health foods" in the meantime, have increased in popularity among athletes. For instance, the late Steve Prefontaine, the American record holder in the 3,000 and 5,000 meter runs, and Ron Jourdan, the 1969 Indoor N.C.A.A. Champion in the high jump, both consumed a breakfast drink that includes wheat germ and brewer's yeast. The assistant track coach for the Bay Area Striders in California recently made a statement concerning the use of "health foods" on his team: "I've obtained good results by giving my athletes ginseng capsules and wheat germ. They seem to cure many minor aches and pains connected with athletics." In addition, many successful weightlifters and shot-putters adhere to the daily rituals of eating such things as organic foods, desiccated liver, lecithin, yogurt, honey, and carrot juice. Naturally these people think that such foods make them bigger, stronger, and healthier.

Do the various "health foods" really work? Some Olympic athletes think not. George Frenn, the American record holder in the hammer throw and former world champion powerlifter has this to say, "I used to take vitamins by injection and eat many health foods, but not anymore. I think they are all a bunch of hooey." Dave Wottle, world record holder and Olympic champion in the 800-meter run, when asked if he consumed any special "health foods" replied, "I don't take anything artificial except Rolaids." The same goes for 110-meter high hurdle champion Rod Milburn as he replied, "I eat no special foods. A lot of hard work is responsible for my winning the gold medal." Jeff Galloway, American record holder for the ten-mile run gives an opinion which seems to summarize the thoughts of many of the Olympic athletes concerning health foods: "I'm a firm believer in three balanced meals a day. Even if there were magic foods or pills available which would make me run faster, I'd rather know that I did it on my own."

What constitutes a "health food?" Actually, the term "health food" is a misnomer. The health of an individual is the result of many factors, one of which is food. The body does not require any particular food, but uses some 50 nutrients in varying amounts. None of the nutrients is considered to be a "health" nutrient, but by definition any nutrient required for human nutrition is essential to life and health even though some are required in only very small amounts. Nevertheless, "health food" stores and the products they sell continue to grow in popularity.

Such growth has occasioned the rise of a number of questions.

What kind of products are sold in "health food" stores? Are they dangerous to use? Are they useful? And if so, are they worth it? Perhaps the best way to discuss these questions is to first of all present a brief history of the development of the so-called "health foods."

HISTORY AND DEVELOPMENT

"Health foods" are as old as mankind. Primitive people frequently believed that what a man ate was what he became. They refused to eat the flesh of the timid deer or the insidious snake, and sought the hearts of lions or other brave animals. Writings before the time of Christ record how Romans thought cabbage was a miracle food. Also among Romans were those who were sure that good health came only with sacrifice, discomfort, self-discipline, and stern attitudes. Among the modern "health food" faddists, this is still a common way of thinking.

Medicine and nutrition progressed little beyond this stage until the sixteenth century. During the sixteenth century many doctors began dissections and chemical trials on humans, which led to the formation of an alchemistic sort of secret to health. Since there was little understanding of human physiology and no sound theory of the origins of disease, the chief method of healing was to feed something unusual or repulsive. Examples of unusual recommendations were worms for lung disease, deer fat for nerves, and goose fat for piles.

Settlers of the New World and later immigrants brought along their ideas on medication. Sometimes notions sprang from a panicky need to discover the reason why. In 1832 when cholera broke out on the eastern seaboard, many cities, among them New York, promptly banned the sale of fruit as fresh fruit was associated with the epidemic. Needless to say, the cholera epidemic continued.

Shortly thereafter, an ordained minister by the name of Sylvester Graham began to lecture on the benefits of vegetables and the evils of meat. He particularly advocated putting the bran back into wheat flour. Graham's ideas spread rapidly as evidenced by the popularity of the now famous "Graham Cracker."

The twentieth century ushered in the health and breakfast cereal ideas of John H. Kellogg and Charles W. Post of Battle Creek, Michigan. Although Kellogg and Post were friends at first, they became bitter competitors and formed separate companies that manufactured their cure-alls. Many of their cereals, e.g., *Kellogg's Corn Flakes* and *Post's Grape Nuts,* are popular today, even though their claims are certainly less extravagant.

With the discovery of various nutrients, particularly the much publicized vitamins, a wave of cures and miracle "health foods" burst onto the American table. As a result, within the last 25 years, "health food" writers have flourished. A few of the best known writers in the field are: Adelle Davis, Jerome I. Rodale, D.C. Jarvis, Robert Cummings, Gayelord Hauser, and Bob Hoffman. Probably the best known writer of this group is the late Adelle Davis. Several of her books have become best sellers, e.g. *Let's Get Well* and *Let's Eat Right to Keep Fit.* She wrote in a very readable and interesting style. However, according to Dr. Fredrick Stare of the Department of Nutrition at Harvard, about half of what Miss Davis wrote makes sense nutritionally and the other half does not. Nevertheless, Miss Davis and the other "health foods" writers have made vast fortunes from their books, food supplements, claims, and cures.

QUESTIONS AND ANSWERS
CONCERNING "HEALTH FOODS"

Question: **What are organically grown fruits and vegetables?**

Answer: "Organically grown" is a term now applied not only to foods raised without chemical fertilizers, but also to foods grown without chemical pesticides. While such foods often cost more than the commercially-grown (supermarket) fruits and vegetables, their nutritional value or nutrient content is not superior or any better.

Actually, there is no way of being certain that foods sold or promoted as "organically grown" were in actual fact grown under those conditions. Frequently, they were not because there just aren't that many growers who refuse to use scientific know-how in their operations. But even if one could be certain that the product was "organically grown," they are not superior to foods grown with fertilizers and pesticides. The United States Department of Agriculture has been unable to find significant differences between the nutritional content of organically grown and ordinary fruits and vegetables.

While we do need to be concerned about the health hazards of DDT and other pesticides, the main harm seems to be to wildlife, not humans. Recently, Dr. Hilda White of Northwestern University noted that if modern agricultural technology were to be discarded in favor of organic farming, the worldwide problems of hunger, malnutrition, and famine would be multiplied immeasurably.

Without chemical fertilizers, farmers would have to use twice as much land to produce the same amount of crops. Secretary of Agriculture Earl Butz has said 50,000,000 people would starve to death if we went back to organic fertilizers entirely. It has been estimated that 80 percent of the foods in our supermarkets would disappear if all pesticides, herbicides, chemical fertilizers, and additives were banned.

Synthetic fertilizers and processed foods have tremendous potential for helping meet the food needs of our rapidly expanding population, but they must both be used with discretion. Soils can be over fertilized reducing crop yield and people can fill their shopping carts with trash foods. Nutrition awareness is an excellent motivator, but it can produce fear, distrust, and a profit bonanza for some; or it can help improve health and vitality, and provide a fair gain for honest businessmen. It all depends on whether people can be taught to apply basic concepts of food and nutrition.

Question: **Is it true that rose hips provide a more nutritious source of vitamin C than synthetic vitamin C tablets?**

Answer: Faddists are quick to promote the vitamins from natural sources as opposed to vitamins that are produced synthetically. However, there are no differences between natural and synthetic vitamins, except for the higher cost of the former.

Actually all foods are mixtures of chemicals. Chemicals are not dangerous or unnatural in themselves. The vitamin C in tablet form is identical with the naturally occurring product. Once the chemical identity of a food or nutrient is known, synthesized and sold, we are taught to distrust it.

Just as every food or nutrient can produce undesirable side effects if consumed in excessive quantities, so can chemicals be used unwisely. Foods or nutrients are just like drugs; they are necessary for health, but they can be abused. Chemical fertilizers can quickly and efficiently restore the nutrient content of deficient soils, but since chemical fertilizers are usually potent and concentrated, they must be used carefully. If used unwisely they may cause nutrient imbalance in soils and therefore poor

130

yield of crops grown on such soil. Soil tests must first be run to determine what particular deficiency exists in the particular soil.

Question: **I've heard that most of our processed food is highly contaminated and most of its nutritional value destroyed. Is that true?**

Answer: All of our foods contain many additives, some of which are unintentional or contaminants and others of which are intentional additives. Additives in foods are used to improve flavor and texture, quality, nutritional content, prolong shelf life, and in the preparation of convenience foods.

The benefits of food additives have been clearly demonstrated again and again. One of the earliest indications of such benefit for the American people came around 1924 with the addition of iodine to table salt. Iodized salt eradicated goiter almost overnight and accounted for a 75 percent decrease in infant mortality rate among people living in the Midwest.

The very serious and often fatal disease pellagra, which plagued many people in the South, was similarly eradicated following the addition of niacin to corn meal and bread. The addition of vitamin D to milk and vitamin B to rice was responsible for greatly reducing the incidence of rickets and beriberi, respectively.

One could also ask where would spice cake, ginger bread, french fried potatoes, and sausage be without additives.

Question: **Should the athlete eat "organic meat and poultry?"**

Answer: This phrase refers mainly to beef, pork and fowl from animals who have never been exposed to hormones, antibiotics, or other drugs. Such chemicals are commonly injected into or fed to livestock and are supposed to be dangerous to man. Again, it is impossible to tell whether such meat has been produced as promoted; it is twice as expensive as the more typical meats; and the United States Department of Agriculture has been unable to substantiate claims that organic meats are safer or more beneficial than non-organic meats.

Question: **I've been eating a wheat germ cereal every morning for years. Should I continue to include it in my diet?**

Answer: Wheat germ is the most nutritious part of the wheat plant and it is often destroyed during the milling of wheat flour. It is a rich source of B vitamins, protein, and vitamin E. Many people enjoy its flavor. For example, when toasted, wheat germ becomes a tasty cereal with a nut-like flavor, or the oil can be used on salads. Some athletes even drink the oil straight from the bottle.

Claims are made that wheat germ can prevent aging, muscular dystrophy, and heart disease. Many athletes also believe that wheat germ oil increases their strength and endurance. But none of these claims that wheat germ is a unique supplier of some essential or therapeutic ingredients have been substantiated by well-controlled studies.

Again the answer is to eat a well-balanced or mixed diet. Wheat germ is not an essential food; it is not unique or magic. Enriched flour, fruits, vegetables, meat, and dairy products as well as many other foods supply the same nutrients found in wheat germ.

Question: **What are fertile eggs? Are they more nutritious than regular eggs?**

Answer: "Fertile eggs," which are supposedly available only at "health food" stores, are promoted as being very special and having a greater nutrient content than infertile or sterile eggs. The implication of the description of "fertile eggs," is that there are infertile eggs being layed by sterile chickens; namely those raised in egg-laying batteries (cages). The claim is that the chicken who is unconfined and allowed to roam about eating insects, scratching in the dirt, etc., is able to lay a better egg. The egg laying capacity of the hen who roams about the farmer's yard is supposed to be superior to the egg-laying capacity of the hen whose diet has been scientifically designed and carefully regulated to be sure she is receiving all the nutrients she needs.

Actually the so called "fertile eggs" should be called "yard eggs" — which may or may not be fertile. Again you can't be sure that eggs sold in "health food" stores are fertile. In order to be sure the egg was fertile, you would have had to allow the hen to mate with a sexually potent rooster, incubate the newly layed egg for 36 hours and then examine it under a high power microscope to determine whether embryonic formation had begun. The truth of the matter is that both fertile and nonfertile eggs have the same nutrients, content of cholesterol and lecithin, poaching characteristics, or you name it. Of course you can pay 40 cents more per dozen for fertile eggs and perhaps this will make them taste about 40 cents better!

Question: **While visiting a California beach last summer, I noticed that many athletes were drinking certified raw milk. Is raw milk better than regular milk?**

Answer: Although certified raw milk may contain somewhat larger amounts of certain nutrients than regular homogenized and pasteurized milk, it is more expensive and dangerous to consume. "Health food" devotees point out that pasteurization destroys most of the beneficial hormones, enzymes, steroids and a large portion of the fat- and water-soluble vitamins in milk. The body is not able to absorb the large enzymes or most of the hormone molecules. Rather, it digests them to smaller molecules, absorbs them and then synthesizes what compounds it needs. Although pasteurization destroys some nutrients in milk, it also kills dangerous bacteria. And that's the whole point of pasteurization. To safely market unpasteurized milk, which is free of dangerous bacteria, would necessitate impeccable hygiene and constant supervision of cows, equipment and employees. The greater ease of processing pasteurized milk as well as safer consumption far outweighs the advantage of supplying a few more nutrients. These lost nutrients can easily be obtained in other foods.

Question: **What is brewer's yeast? Is it a desirable constituent of an athlete's diet?**

Answer: Brewer's yeast is a bitter, yellow powder that is related to a variety of yeast that is a by-product of beer brewing. Thus, it is actually misnamed "brewer's" yeast. It does, however, contain large amounts of B vitamins, amino acids, and minerals. Supplementing the diet with dried brewer's yeast might be useful if you are deficient in protein and B vitamins; but eating bitter yeast isn't the most efficient or the most appetizing way to obtain these nutrients. Besides, only vitamins obtainable by prescription contain B vitamins in high enough dosages to be therapeutically valuable.

Question: **Is raw sugar better for me than regular table sugar?**

Answer: Real raw sugar is illegal to sell in the United States since it is unsanitary. What is actually sold under this name is a partially refined cane sugar. Raw sugar has a few more minerals than regular sugar but not enough to justify its higher price. Furthermore, most Americans eat more sugar than they should, or is healthy, since it unbalances the diet so easily in favor of calories. The problem is not the wrong kind of sugar in the diet, but the consumption of too many calories.

Question: **What about black strap molasses? I've heard it's a cure for many ailments?**
Answer: This thick syrup is the residue after sugar cane is refined into white sugar. Unlike honey and table sugar, which provide only empty calories, black strap molasses does contain calcium, iron, and most of the B vitamins. However, claims that black strap molasses can prevent cancer, cure ulcers, varicose veins, arthritis, or any other trouble have not been authenticated and should be looked upon with considerable skepticism.

Question: **Will yogurt help me digest my food more completely?**
Answer: Yogurt is a fermented milk product and like all dairy products, it is an excellent source of protein and calcium. Since most supermarkets have been carrying yogurt since the early 1960's, only the very unusual forms are sold in "health food" stores. Their prices are usually double the cost of most grocery store varieties. Yogurt was once thought to assist intestinal function by providing certain beneficial bacteria. However, control of the intestinal bacteria has been shown not to be very critical nor dependent upon the intake of yogurt. Yogurt has the same nutritional value as buttermilk, which is considerably less expensive.

Question: **What is the difference between the untreated vegetable oils sold in "health food" stores and regular vegetable oils?**
Answer: These untreated oils (cold pressed from such plants as safflower, corn, cotton, and soy bean) are bottled without preservatives or additives. Taken in the proper amounts, these oils can provide a valuable source of polyunsaturated fatty acids in your diet. However, the nutritional value of the vegetable oils is easily destroyed when left to stand, or when heated. All untreated oils must be purchased in small quantities and not

heated for they are extremely perishable. Furthermore, the Department of Agriculture has been unable to find any harmful effects that are produced from using the common vegetable oils that do contain preservatives.

Question: **Would a desiccated liver supplement be helpful to the athlete trying to improve his endurance?**

Answer: Desiccated liver, in pill or powder form is a good source of vitamin B_{12}. Vitamin B_{12} is vital for protection against pernicious anemia, which results in weakness and loss of energy and endurance. Therefore, faddists reasoned that if desiccated liver would keep you from getting weak and rundown from anemia, it also would aid in developing endurance. As a result, some athletes have been known to have taken desiccated liver tablets by the handfuls.

Actually pernicious anemia is a very rare condition occurring in those who eat a total vegetarian diet, or who have had their stomach totally removed, or those who have a genetic problem and can't absorb the vitamin B_{12} in their diet. Desiccated liver probably wouldn't help the latter group because they couldn't absorb the vitamin B_{12} in it. Intramuscular injections of the vitamin or a preparation to improve absorption are usually given.

Question: **Will lecithin keep men from having heart attacks?**

Answer: Lecithin is the natural emulsifier found in egg yolks and soybeans and is sold in capsule and powder form at "health food" stores. It has long been publicized in health magazines as an antidote to high blood cholesterol and heart disease. Evidence shows that lecithin cannot dissolve the plaques in the blood vessels that contribute to heart attacks. Unfortunately, solving the problems associated with high blood cholesterol concentrations and heart attacks are much more complex than a simple feeding of lecithin to the patient.

Question: **I've been drinking several glasses of raw vegetable juices each day. Are they necessary?**

Answer: Carrot juice and other vegetable juices have been promoted using the rationale that the vitamins and minerals contained in these vegetables are essential nutrients and "if a little is good, more is better." In moderate amounts, these juices

135

are not likely to hurt anyone and most of them are quite appealing to the taste buds. Raw vegetable juices, however, are costly and the large amounts frequently recommended may provide excessive amounts of liquids and sodium in the diet. Furthermore, the whole fruit or vegetable contributes desirable residue or fiber, which is necessary for normal gastrointestinal function and regularity.

Question: **What is brown rice?**
Answer: Brown rice is just ordinary rice that has not had its outer layers of husk and embryo removed by polishing. It does contain more protein and vitamins than unenriched white rice, but, the difference is small enough to be unimportant unless rice forms a major portion of your diet. Some extremists advocate eating practically nothing but brown rice and other grains — a diet that is grossly deficient in many nutrients and even dangerous. Several people have in fact starved to death following such a diet.

Question: **I'm amazed at the number of exotic foods that are sold in "health food" stores. What advice can you give me concerning these obscure foods?**
Answer: Many people are becoming interested in exotic foods. Should sesame seeds be on your dining room table, or garlic oil in your pantry? Will avocado oil clear your complexion? Which tea is best for health — buckthorn, mullein leaf, slippery elm, wormwood, or sassafras? These exotic products go on and on. And each product is supposed to provide a specific benefit for health, according to the faddist.

Medical authorities and nutrition scientists who aren't earning a living from the sale of "health foods" seem to agree on answers to these questions. Stay away from exotic and obscure food products, unless you know exactly what they are and what they will do to you; and don't be afraid to seek professional advice when questions or problems arise.

DISCUSSION

Although these and many other "health food" claims have also been disproved, they are still promoted as *new* and *miraculous* to a growing body of misinformed buyers. Who are these misinformed buyers? According to James Trager, three basic groups are interested in "health foods": (1) people motivated by a simple desire for good food, (2) people concerned about environmental decay from persistent chemical pesticides and herbicides, and (3) people who have anxieties about their appearance and physical well-being, which they link to what they eat. The third group, which by the way includes many athletes, is by far the largest of the three.

Members of these groups frequently testify that they feel just "wonderful" as a result of eating this food or taking that pill. The alleged benefit of "health foods" may be in the *faith* that the buyer puts in these foods. This psychological benefit or "placebo effect" should not be sold short.

No doubt much of the faith in "health foods" is developed from the positive encouragement of the so-called "Nutrition Counselor" behind the cash register. Such counselors thrive because customers need them. Ignorant consumers cry for positive advice and remedies to their problems. The danger in this advice lies in the fact that most of the nutrition counselors are self-trained and have no formal background in nutrition or medicine. Yet, they dispense information that the customer takes as the gospel truth! Most of this advice is simply ridiculous and unjustified. "How to succeed without trying" seems to be the cry of most people in trouble and they are eager to believe any promise of cure, no matter how ridiculous it may sound, if it doesn't demand self-discipline or a change in habits upon which they have become dependent.

Often people with nutrient deficiencies or unusual nutrient requirements can not be safely self-diagnosed or self-treated. Pills should not be substituted for meals. Furthermore, it is difficult for the layman who is searching for an answer to tell the difference between useful recommendations and the sales pitch of a product. You may waste money taking unprescribed vitamins and mineral supplements and do yourself no harm, since the excess is usually excreted. However, overdoses of vitamins A and D can be harmful and the prolonged intake of excessive amount of energy sources; protein, and various minerals can produce serious damage to health and well-being.

It is true that the average American diet has declined in nutritive value over the last 20 years. This decline is partly related to the plentifulness of sugar and our susceptibility to convenience foods (e.g., TV dinners). But, these undesirable eating habits can be improved without "health foods" or diet supplements.

To summarize, the products sold in "health food" stores are not more nutritious than products sold at your local supermarket. In fact they're much more expensive and it's often difficult to be certain you're getting what you're paying for. Don't be misled about the power of "health foods." Stick to a well-balanced diet and you'll have plenty of vim and vigor!

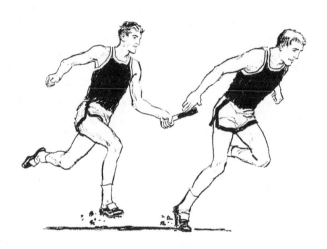

9

Turn On or Off
With Drugs

DRUGS AREN'T classified as foods, although many times they are taken by mouth and thought of in a similar fashion by numerous athletes. Foods would be defined as anything that is taken into the body through the alimentary canal in order to supply nutrients to meet the physiological requirements of cells and/or the psychological and sociological needs of man. During special situations materials not generally considered foods may be desirable sources of nutrients or therapeutic agents, for example the intravenous administration of glucose. Various other materials such as drugs, alcohol, and tobacco are often consumed without medical prescription. These can't be recommended because they don't serve as a safe or satisfactory source of the nutrients they provide. Plus, they can contribute hazardous side effects. Some of these materials will be considered in this chapter, however, because of their widespread usage among athletes and the false claims associated with them.

The use of drugs to improve performance in sports has plagued coaches and trainers for many years. How widespread drug usage is among athletes is impossible to state other than by certain educated guesses. *Sports Illustrated* recently stated that some players on all the professional football teams have used various drugs in hopes of improving their performance. Former major league pitcher, Jim Bouton, in his book *Ball Four,* made the statement that he felt as many as 40 percent of major league baseball players used "bennies."

139

A former college track coach, Tom Ecker, goes as far as to state that, "it's a great rarity today for someone to achieve athletic success who doesn't take drugs." Jack Scott, controversial writer and director of the Institute for the Study of Sports and Society, observed at the 1968 Olympic Games in Mexico City that:

> Athletes and coaches were not involved in debating the morality or propriety of taking drugs. The only debate was over which drugs were most effective and what kinds of amphetamines could go undetected in the tests Olympic officials were requiring athletes to take at the conclusion of their competition.

Evidently the drug scene is slowly developing into mammoth proportions. Not only are drugs frequently used by college and professional athletes, but certain high school players regularly take them as well as some of the kids in the pee wee leagues. There have also been several fatalities among athletes involved with drugs. Danish cyclist, Knut Jensen, collapsed and died at the 1960 Olympic Games in Rome after a fatal dose of amphetamines and nicotinic acid compound was given to him by his trainer. In addition, Dick Howard, bronze medal winner in the 400-meter hurdles at Rome, died of an overdose of drugs. And more recently there occurred the case of the British cyclist Simpson who, after taking amphetamines, collapsed and died after a race. Apparently several fatalities were required in order to make the public understand the urgency of the problem.

It is important that coaches and athletes be aware of the various facts and fallacies concerning drugs and athletic performance. This chapter will discuss some of the functions and dangers of different drugs that have been used by athletes, and present questions and answers pertaining to drug usage among athletes.

FUNCTION AND SIDE EFFECTS

A drug is broadly defined as any chemical agent that has a measurable effect on a living organism. However, most laymen relate the use of drugs to the prevention and cure of a specific disease. Unfortunately the use of drugs by athletes seems to depend on whether or not the substance is believed effective or is habit-forming. If the drug isn't a stimulant, its use apparently doesn't conflict with the rules on doping of the Amateur Athletic Union, at least as interpreted by many athletes. Of course some people would argue that the athletes' definition of "stimulant" and "habit-forming" has been stretched to meet his own needs and wants. Many athletes also confuse habit-forming with addiction. Few athletes are addicts, but drug usage has become a habit as far as some athletes' dependence on them is concerned. A large majority of the drugs taken by athletes are habit-forming, often producing undesirable or dangerous side effects.

Most of the drugs that are used by athletes can be classified into five categories: (1) central nervous system depressants and stimulants, (2) drugs acting on autonomic effector cells, (3) cardiovascular drugs, (4) androgenic-anabolic steroids, and (5) restorative drugs.

Central Nervous System
Depressants and Stimulants

The central nervous system depressant that most people are familiar is alcohol. Although seldom used by athletes in hopes that it will improve performance, alcohol's effect on performance should be determined since it is frequently consumed by athletes. The initial stimulation from alcohol results from the unrestrained activity of the lower centers of the brain that are freed of suppression by the higher inhibitory control mechanisms. Alcohol increases neither mental nor physical ability. There is a minor effect on respiration, circulation, and skeletal muscle activity, but the amount of work performed may be increased due to a decreased feeling (or perception) of fatigue. The late Dr. Peter V. Karpovich of Springfield College, in his book, *Physiology of Muscular Activity,* further notes that alcohol has a harmful effect on speed in swimming or running short distances.

Central nervous system stimulants that have been used by athletes include caffeine, camphor, cocaine, coramine, strychnine, and metrazol. Amphetamine also stimulates the brain directly but is classified with the drugs that act on the autonomic effector cells. Of the central nervous system stimulants, caffeine and cocaine are the most commonly and widely used.

Caffeine is a relatively potent stimulant that produces a keener appreciation of sensory stimuli, increases motor activity, decreases reaction time, and retards the feeling of fatigue. Central stimulation is responsible for the increased capacity for work in that the perception of fatigue is prevented. Again Dr.

141

Karpovich found that caffeine increased work output but doesn't affect speed in running short distances.

Cocaine has the capacity to increase muscular work, and this too, is primarily due to a lessened awareness of fatigue. Heart rate is increased after moderate doses because of increased central and peripheral sympathetic stimulation. Several studies with cocaine have shown that it slightly increases endurance and the speed of recovery after bicycle riding.

Drugs Acting on Autonomic Effector Cells

Certain drugs can imitate the effect of nerve stimulation on muscles or glands. The most popular of these drugs are amphetamine, epinephrine, and nicotine.

Amphetamine drugs are widely used by athletes. The most common brands of these "pep pills" are Dexedrine, Benzedrine, Syndrox, and Ritalin. Amphetamine stimulates the respiratory and arousal mechanisms of the brain as well as the central nervous system. There is also an inconsistent stimulation of blood pressure.

Former professional football player Alex Karras notes that the use of "pep pills" depends largely upon how the team is doing. Teams that are winning or have inspirational coaches might not need drugs to "get up" for the game, while other players need pills to perform regardless of how well the team is doing. Some players have tried amphetamines and found that they perform better without them. Thus, the effects of amphetamines on physical performance are varied as much depends on the fatigue, personality, motivation, and sustained attention of the one taking the drug.

Epinephrine also acts directly on the effector cells of the body, but it has very little effect on the central nervous system. Oxygen consumption is increased, blood sugar and lactic acid levels are elevated, and the glycogen content of the liver and muscles is decreased. Laboratory work with epinephrine, in animals and man, has shown that the drug doesn't produce an increase in performance capacity, although it does make the subjects feel more energetic.

Nicotine, the active principle of tobacco, inhibits skeletal muscle on the basis of reducing the amount of oxygen that the blood can carry or transport. However, the use of tobacco exhibits predictable but often multiple changes in athletes. Most authorities tend to agree that smoking can hinder neuromuscular and cardiovascular performance.

Cardiovascular Drugs

Certain cardiovascular drugs have been used by athletes, especially cyclists, to improve performance. Included in this group are Thiocyanate, Rauwalfia, Hydralazine, and Khellan. There have been few controlled scientific studies regarding their effect on work performance in normal subjects. Nevertheless, you should realize that most of the cardiovascular drugs are extremely potent, and the death of several athletes has been attributed to their use.

Androgenic-Anabolic Steroids

The most popular drugs used at the present time by athletes are the androgenic-anabolic steroids. *Anabolic* relates to nitrogen retention and protein building, while *androgenic* refers to the production of masculine characteristics. These drugs are synthetic forms of testosterone and other male hormones. A few of the most common brand names are Dianabol, Winstrol, Anavar, Nilevar, Durabolin, and Methyltestosterone. In males it is presumed that the presence of androgens in increased quantities contributes to greater strength and muscle mass.

Several studies investigating the effect of androgenic-anabolic steroids on strength and performance have produced conflicting results. Many subtle factors may account for these differences. The type and degree of response to steroid drugs depends a great deal on the age of the subject. Thus increased muscle strength occurs to a greater extent when the drugs are given before puberty or after age 50, primarily because of the decreased production of testosterone in the body. Another important factor has to do with amount and regularity of the drug dosage. For example, the maximum recommended dosage of Dianabol is 10 to 20 mg. per day for three months. Yet many athletes consume two to three times that amount for as long as a year. These reasons probably explain much of the difference between statements concerning the effects of such drugs increasing strength.

Recently, a physician at a large New York hospital examined over 300 athletes who had been consuming large amounts of steroid drugs. He emphatically stated that he could detect clinical damage in 100 percent of the athletes up to six months after the drugs were discontinued, and permanent damage in more than 25 percent of the athletes. In his opinion, these drugs cannot improve the physical performance of a healthy, mature athlete.

Restorative Drugs

Restorative drugs can be grouped under two categories: relaxants and pain killers.

Relaxant drugs include sedatives, sleeping pills, barbiturates, tranquilizers, and muscle relaxers. These drugs have been used in most sports to prevent cramps, tension, and tightness of muscles. Unlike the other drugs, relaxants aren't used secretly in most sports. No one contends that these drugs increase performance potential beyond normal limits. In fact it is generally conceded that they dull a performer's senses. However, the relaxant drugs might be of benefit in some sports like golf.

The anti-pain drugs are of two types: those that provide local anesthetic action for aches and strains, and those that are also anti-inflammatory. The first type includes: Novocain (procaine HCL) and Xylocaine (lidocaine), which are usually given by injection; ethyl chloride, which is sprayed on; and those that begin with aspirin and work up to include opiates, which act on the central nervous center. Drugs such as Novocain numb the nerve endings and deaden pain in injured sections of the body where they're injected. But this practice is considered risky because an athlete can reinjure himself seriously without knowing it.

The second type of pain killers are the potent anti-inflammatory drugs such as Cortisone, phenylbutazone, and the once banned dimenthyl sulfoxide (DMSO). Cortisone, a synthetic form of an adrenal-gland hormone, is often injected into inflamed joints, tendons, and muscles. Although frequent injections of Cortisone can temporarily eliminate pain, at the same time it can impede healing and produce undesirable side reactions of a very severe nature. This is not an uncommon occurence when the drug is injected into the elbow joints of baseball players and tennis players.

QUESTIONS AND ANSWERS CONCERNING DRUGS AND ATHLETIC PERFORMANCE

Question: **Why do so many athletes take drugs?**

Answer: Several factors contribute to the current drug problem in athletics. Drugs of all kinds are prevalent in the American culture today as evidenced by the many young people who smoke marijuana and experiment with hallucinatory drugs. Most of the drugs discussed in this book are readily available to the athlete on the "black market" or even legitimately through the proper channels. Even more important than this is the incredible pressure on coaches and athletes to win at all costs. Coaches and athletes are frequently reminded of the late Vince Lombardi's philosophy: "Winning is not everything. It is the only thing." Therefore, in their frantic search for victory, athletes many times are forced to turn to drugs because they know their competitors are using them or because they believe they are important if not essential to winning.

Added to these reasons is the fact that athletes are some of the world's worst faddists. Numerous athletes swear by certain rituals, numbers, modes of dress, words, coins, and bits of magic. Perhaps more than any other group, their reputation and salary depend on environmental conditions and luck. Therefore, it is understandable why so many athletes are prone to experiment with any available drug. The athlete's foremost dream is that somewhere there is a pill that will automatically make or help him become a champion overnight.

A most interesting study concerning drugs has been going on in France and was reported by Dr. Donald Cooper in an issue of the *Journal of the American Medical Association* (August 28, 1972). For the last five years, French scientists have tested almost all of the drugs previously accused of being used in the doping of horses. Thoroughbred race horses have been run in every conceivable way — with drugs, without drugs, warmed up, not warmed up, rested, and fatigued. Surprisingly enough, they have not been able to demonstrate in any way that any drug can make a horse run faster or consistently improve its performance. These findings seem to point out that horses don't benefit from the so called "placebo power," while many humans do. However, the danger with certain drugs is that they can mask fatigue. Under these conditions, an athlete or a race horse may run past normal capacity and when combined with heat buildup, may cause circulatory failure. But, this does not mean that the athlete or the horse can go any faster!

Question: **Are drugs more apt to be consumed by participants in one particular sport group as opposed to others?**

Answer: No one particular group has a monopoly on drug usage. However, participants in certain sports seem to be notorious drug users. Among the most prevalent users of drugs in the United States are the *weightlifters,* a group that includes Olympic lifters, powerlifters, and body builders. Running a close second to weightlifters would probably be trackmen, particularly those who participate in the strength events such as the shot-put and discus. It has been estimated by certain authorities that 80 percent of the weightlifters, shot-putters, discus throwers, and javelin throwers are using some type of drugs.

There are several reasons why weightlifters and trackmen are so drug prone. Both compete as individuals, a fact that naturally makes them more introspective. Much time is spent by these athletes in watching their body weight, food intake, muscle tone, skin tone, bruises, and strains. Thus, weightlifters and trackmen are especially susceptible to any suggestion that there may be some secret drug that will improve their strength, muscle size, or endurance. And, too, many of these athletes compete in other countries, where they are able to hear about and obtain the latest foreign drugs.

Question: **Are androgenic-anabolic steroid drugs safe to use by athletes? Are there any side effects?**

Answer: A similar question was recently answered by Dr. Alexander J. Graziano of CIBA Pharmaceutical Company concerning their steroid drug Dianabol:

> The use of Dianabol in healthy males between the ages of 15 and 18 years is not well-documented. There would seem to be no contraindication to short courses of therapy using recommended doses as long as epiphyses are closed, but we here at CIBA cannot sanction its use. From time to time we hear of its use by football teams and weightlifters without side effects; but, again, these are not controlled studies. In general, the use of drugs of any kind for the

expected improvements of athletic endeavor seems to be frowned upon.

Dr. Graziano continues by saying:

The American Medical Association has officially recommended that athletes not use oral anabolic agents, all of which are related to methyltestosterone, as an artificial aid in building muscles. The best way to excel in athletics is to have proper nutrition and graded exercise in order to build athletic proficiency without any artificial stimulus. Under the circumstances, our company can in no way recommend the use of Dianabol in athletes for improved performance.

The AMA has also listed certain adverse reactions and precautions for anyone using these hormones. Among the side reactions are nausea, edema, signs of virilization, acne, and deepening of the voice. Most of these changes are irreversible and apply to women as well as men.

Question: **What opinions do coaches and team physicians have concerning drug usage among athletes?**

Answer: Some authorities think that drugs were first introduced to the American athlete by coaches, trainers, and team physicians from high school through the professional ranks. There are frequent stories of how assistant coaches slipped pep pills to certain players before each game. But, while most coaches probably don't slip pills to their players, they often turn their heads while the players take their own pills and pretend to be unaware of drug usage.

Dr. H. Kay Dooley, director of the Wood Memorial Clinic in Pomona, California, openly supports the use of drugs in athletic performance. He believes that medically supervised drug usage by athletes presents no danger to either athletes or the sport itself.

A similar view is also taken by Bill Starr, former managing editor of a physical fitness-weightlifting journal (*Strength and Health*). He says:

I do believe that anabolics are safe when used properly and that they do result in a substantial strength gain. I believe that amphetamines do bring positive results to some lifters and are not harmful when used properly. And I do believe it is the right of the individual to choose whether to use these substances or not.

Some physicians take an opposing view of this issue. One such physician is Dr. Robert Kerlan of the Los Angeles Lakers basketball team. Dr. Kerlan believes that someone should speak out strongly against most drug usage. There are valid medical reasons for prescribing drugs for athletes in some situations, notes Kerlan. However, he is quick to point out that the excessive and secretive use of drugs is likely to eventually become a major athletic scandal which will shake the public's confidence in many sports. Therefore, when athletes start using drugs to gain an unnatural advantage, the purpose of sports as well as the individuals involved in such practices becomes corrupted.

Question: **What can be done to control the drug usage in athletics?**

Answer: This is a complex and difficult question to answer. Bill Gilbert, writing in *Sports Illustrated* (July 7, 1969), recommends that authorities look to the sport of horseracing for guidelines in dealing with the drug problems. Although horseracing doesn't deal with human subjects, it is the one major American sport which has drug regulations. Racing officials have admitted that drugs can affect racing performance; they have defined what drugging is and established an apparatus to detect the practice and punish the offenders.

It is interesting to note that some positive steps have been taken by the International Olympic Committee Medical Commission. In the 1968 Olympic Games in Mexico City, some limited testing was done among the athletes, but few rules and regulations had been standardized. However, during the 1972 Olympics, most of the doping rules had been standardized and the procedures perfected. Therefore, urine samples from over 1,000 of the 8,000 competing athletes were collected and analyzed for the misuse of drugs. The results revealed at least 23 positive tests with some of those being medal winners. So, some steps and controls are being taken.

Former athlete and coach, Jack Scott, also has some positive recommendations. "If sports were to return to the old-fashioned but still relevant philosophy that 'it's not important if you win or lose, but how you play the game,' drug usage would certainly be attenuated, if not eliminated." However, Scott is probably correct in his pessimistic hope for this possibility as when he states: "as long as there is inordinate emphasis on winning, athletes will continue using drugs or any other aid they believe will contribute to the likelihood of victory."

Since there have been very few well-controlled studies concerning the effects and side reactions of drug usage by athletes, it would appear that a fair settlement of the issue would include more national and international rules and regulations and a better means of enforcing them.

In closing this chapter, I can't help but remember what strength-training expert, Arthur Jones, perhaps one of the few remaining "let's get back to logic" thinkers, told me recently concerning drugs and athletic performance:

> There is no known drug that will improve the performance of a healthy individual . . . and there never will be such a drug; normal health being just that, normal . . . super health by definition, being impossible.

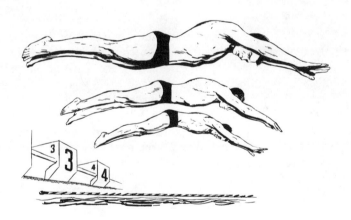

10

Food and Exercise for the Female Athlete

THERE HAS BEEN phenomenal growth of girls' and women's participation in sports during the 1970's. National Federation figures recently released set high school girls' participation in interscholastic sports during the 1974-75 academic year at 1,300,169. That's 342 percent more girls than during the 1970-71 academic year. The most current NCAA report on women's participation in intercollegiate athletic programs shows 31,852 college women engaged in 24 sports. Five years before, only half that many women participated.

But that's just a start. Women of all ages, pre-teens to grandmas, are participating in more organized and unorganized sports than ever before. From archery to weightlifting, from baseball to yachting, you name it and women are getting involved. Newspapers, magazines, and TV are even doing their parts by giving better coverage to women's local and national sporting events.

Where will it all peak? There's no telling because no one knows what impact the Department of Health, Education, and Welfare's Title IX directives (equal funding for men's and women's athletics) will have on the already skyrocketing growth of schoolgirl sports.

This acceleration of women's sports participation, however, is not without problems ... many of which center around such areas as exercise, training, diet, and nutrition. And right or wrong (mostly wrong in my opinion), they seek answers from their big brothers — men's athletics. So . . . that opens the door for all the old myths, misconceptions, and false beliefs that have been floating around men's locker rooms over the last 75 years.

You can save yourself a lot of problems, if you'll *remember* what a wise person once told me:

> *You cannot learn the proper method for training a race horse by asking a race horse.* Instead, try to understand the basic factors involved — and when you do, then you can at least base your training on facts, instead of on well-meant but faulty opinions.

Although the concepts that I've covered in the previous chapters apply, in most instances, to both men and women, this chapter will deal specifically with the female athlete. Let's begin by clearing the ground of certain "old wives' tales," or to be more exact, "old men's locker room tales."

EXERCISE AND LARGE MUSCLES

Most women firmly believe that if they participate in heavy exercise they'll develop large, unfeminine muscles. The truth of the matter is that it's virtually impossible for most women to develop large muscles.

It's no accident that men develop a larger, more defined muscle mass. The effect is the direct result of the male hormone, testosterone, upon the growth mechanism of the male's body.

Before puberty there's little difference between the muscular size and strength of boys and girls. With the onset of puberty, testosterone from the boy's testes and estrogen from the girl's ovaries enter the blood stream, and trigger the development of the appropriate secondary sexual characteristics. Thus, it takes a certain amount of testosterone within the blood stream to influence muscular growth.

There are a small percentage of women who have large muscles, particularly in their legs. These larger than average muscles were either inherited or are the result of an above average amount of testosterone in the system.

The adrenal glands and the sex glands, within both men and women, secrete a small amount of the nondominant hormone. As a result, there are a few women who have inherited larger than average muscles and at the same time have an extra amount of testosterone in their system. These women do have the potential to develop larger than average muscles. (There are also men who have an extra amount of estrogen in their sys-

151

tems, which tends to give them a feminine-like appearance.)

Generally speaking, 99 percent of American women couldn't develop large muscles if their lives depended on it. But heavy exercise is worthwhile because it strengthens and conditions your muscles . . . which in turn will make you a better athlete.

Somewhat related to the above misconception is the idea that women are inferior to men in muscular strength.

STRENGTH: WOMEN VS. MEN

This topic was recently studied by Drs. C. Harmon Brown and Jack H. Wilmore of the University of California at Davis. They placed 47 untrained college-aged women and 26 untrained college-aged men on a 10-week weight training program.

After the program was over, both groups had made substantial gains in strength. In terms of actual weight lifted the upper body strength of the men was 50 percent higher than the women and the lower body strength of the men was 25 percent higher. However, when they figured leg strength relative to lean body weight (total weight minus the weight of fat) the females rated 5.8 percent stronger than the males.

In the final analysis, Dr. Wilmore concludes: " . . . if you look at strength in terms of the size of the individual — minus fat — you find that the strength potential is theoretically similar for both men and women."

Let's move on to the idea that strong muscles make you less flexible, or "muscle bound."

LACK OF FLEXIBILITY

Flexibility is related to your ability to stretch and contract your muscles throughout a full range of movement. Over 434 skeletal muscles are responsible for your overall movement potential.

Muscles were tailor-made to be used. And the "use or lose it" maxim applies nowhere as cogently as here. You can actually lose some of the range of motion of a particular muscle if it isn't used throughout its full stretching and contracting process. In other words, you become "muscle bound" from using your muscles *too little,* not too much. This can be easily observed in the inflexible walk or shuffle that many elderly people develop.

Proper exercise programs apply resistance to your muscles as they are stretched and contracted. So, muscles that have been conditioned in the proper manner are not only strong — but flexible. This was demonstrated in 1975 by Dr. Jim Peterson of the U.S. Military Academy in testing cadets before and after a six-week strength-training program.

As an added attraction, when you increase the strength of a muscle you also increase the *power to weight* ratio, which means that your speed of movement will be improved. In other words: *you'll be faster*.

Speed of movement also relates to the amount of fat that you have on your body. Fat between muscle fibers acts as a friction brake and can actually impede the normal, relatively friction-less contraction of lean muscle fibers. Therefore, it's important to understand the difference between muscle and fat.

COMPOSITION OF MUSCLE AND FAT

You hear it all the time: "If you quit training, your muscles will turn to fat." It's physiologically impossible for muscle to turn to fat. Apparently many people think muscle and fat are the same thing.

Muscle and fat are related in that both contain water, lipids (fats), and protein. The composition, however, is very different. A pound of fat has 3,500 calories while a pound of muscle contains only 600 calories. Most of muscle is water, whereas fatty tissue is mainly composed of fat. The density of muscle is much greater than fat.

Athletes, with high levels of muscular strength, who suddenly quit training, get significant reductions (atrophy) in muscle mass as well as reduction in overall caloric requirements. Thus the athlete who stops training should reduce her caloric intake accordingly. If this isn't done, then what usually occurs is a slow increase in the percentage of body fat and a decrease in the percentage of muscle mass — even though her bodyweight may remain relatively stable.

BODILY FAT DISTRIBTUION

While energy balance (intake vs. output) determines the amount of fat present, other factors determine the way in which it's distributed over your body. The most important of these is *inherited*. Just as different families and different races have characteristic heights, coloring, and nose shapes, they may have characteristic patterns of fat distribution.

Perhaps the best known racial variant is that of the African Hottentot and Bushman. If the women become obese, the bulk of the fat is deposited as a great mound around the buttocks. The mound may actually grow to the size of a large watermelon while the woman remains relatively lean over the rest of her body.

Hormones also influence the distribution of body fat. Androgens and estrogens are largely responsible for the differences in the way men and women deposit fat. The breasts, for example, are mostly fat, not glandular tissue as many people imagine, and estrogens are particularly responsible for this fat deposition.

Generally speaking, as women get older, they tend to deposit fat around their hips and thighs, while men are more likely to deposit it in the abdomen and as a roll around the sides.

EXERCISE AND FAT REDUCTION

Most people believe that concentrated exercise for a particular body part that is laden with fat will be effective in removing the fat (spot reduction). Although exercise does play a role in the reduction of body fat (along with a proper diet), fat is mobilized out of multiple fat cells all over the body. Thus, spot reducing is impossible.

In order to reduce your percentage of body fat, you have to force your body to burn its own fat as a source of energy. Consuming 1,000 less calories a day than your maintenance level will require your body to burn several pounds of fat a week as a source of energy. But even then, the fat will come from all over your body, not just one spot.

Remember, the areas and the order in which you store and lose fat have been genetically determined. Try as you may, you can't change it. But even so, proper exercise will benefit you. Not only will it strengthen your muscles, but the fat and skin that surround these muscles will become tighter and firmer.

Let's now examine some of the most frequently asked questions that women coaches and athletes have about food and exercise. Based on the latest government data and information from other qualified sources, the answers should provide you with some valuable knowledge.

QUESTIONS AND ANSWERS ABOUT
FOOD AND EXERCISE FOR THE FEMALE ATHLETE

Question: **What is energy and where does it come from?**
Answer: Energy is the internal power you must have for everything you do. That's right . . . *everything* . . . from breathing to moving, from digesting to sleeping, even expressing joy or anger.

The sun is our source of energy. In high school we learned that *energy could not be created or destroyed* . . . and it's still true. We can only change its form and the place where it is available.

Only plants have the ability to grow by combining the energy from the sun with the elements from the air and soil and water. Animals get their energy originally from plants . . . and we get our energy from plants *and* animals. From a nutritional viewpoint, food and energy are measured in *calories*.

Question: **How many calories do female athletes 12-18 years of age need a day?**
Answer: The number of calories your athletes need a day depends basically on their age, size, and activity. As a general rule of thumb, your athletes can get an idea of their daily caloric needs by using the following figures:

Age	12-14 years	14-16 years	16-18 years
Suggested calories per pound per day	24 calories	21 calories	19 calories

For example, if Karen is 15 and weighs 114 pounds, she needs about 2,400 calories (114 x 21 = 2,400) a day to supply her energy and growth needs. Of course, these aren't rigid guidelines. More or less active girls will need to adjust their calories per pound accordingly.

Question: **What type foods should be eaten daily by female athletes?**
Answer: The foods that they should eat daily are classified into four basic groups:
2 or more servings from the *meat group,*
4 cups of *dairy products,*
4 or more servings of *vegetables and fruits,*
4 or more servings of *breads and cereals,*

155

Plus, *other foods* (butter, margarine, oils, sugar, and sweets) to complete meals and to provide additional energy.

Varied selections from these *four basic food groups* form the backbone of what nutritionists call a *balanced diet*. These guidelines have received firm support from the American Medical Association for the last 20 years.

Question: **As a coach, what habits should I encourage to derive the best physical performances from my teenage athletes?**

Answer: If your teenage athletes are eager eaters, you worry that they're eating the wrong things. If they're meager eaters, you worry about malnutrition. Either way, you worry that inconsistent eating habits will affect their performances on the athletic field. Unfortunately, you could be right!

Teenage girls are notoriously weight-conscious. In their efforts to stay trim, they've probably developed the poorest eating habits of all age groups. Even girls who know the rules of the eating game often choose to ignore them.

You can do your part by challenging each of your athletes to assume personal responsibility for a year-round schedule of regular exercise, sleep, and well-balanced meals. Encourage your teenage girls to eat more vegetables, especially the green leafy ones, as they are usually neglected. And, *insist* that your athletes eat breakfast.

Question: **Why is breakfast such an important meal?**

Answer: Studies have shown that many teenage girls are listless and inattentive during morning class hours because of poor breakfasts. In one study, of those girls who had poor breakfasts, only one in five ended the day with an adequate diet.

If left to their own devices to choose breakfast food, girls tend to choose poorly, accordingly to a University of California study. Help your girls learn to like breakfast by encouraging them to eat a wide variety of foods.

Examples of nutritious breakfasts are as follows:

1. ¼ cantaloupe
2. 2 ounces of tuna fish salad
3. 2 slices of toast with margarine
4. 1 glass of skim milk

1. Fresh orange or grapefruit sections
2. Peanut butter and banana sandwich
3. 1 scrambled egg
4. 1 glass of skim milk

Question: **Are there scientific reasons why teenage girls are less well nourished than boys?**

Answer: Yes there are. Teenage girls need almost as much protein, vitamins, and minerals as do teenage boys. But they require, and usually wish to eat, only two-thirds to three-fourths of the quantity eaten by boys. Therefore, to eat well, they must choose more carefully. Also, menstruation increases their need for protein and iron. One *cultural* reason for poor diets among teenage girls is a concern with overweight, and an unrealistic ideal of what their figures ought to be like. A teenage girl who can model fashions is probably a nutritional question-mark!

Question: **Should special types and amounts of food be served for a pre-game meal?**

Answer: The meal before any sporting event should be acceptable to the individual athlete. Whatever the athlete feels will help her performance should be eaten.

Question: **Does the pre-game meal supply all the energy needed for a game?**

Answer: No. In fact, the pre-game meal for 98 percent of the female athletes supplies very little of the actual energy that is used in the game. This energy ordinarily comes from food consumed from two to fourteen days prior to the contest.

The only exceptions to this rule are the athletes that participate in continuous activities that last at least 45 minutes ... like long-distance running. Pre-contest meals made up of carbohydrate-rich foods can definitely supply additional energy to these athletes. A carbohydrate-rich meal might include dried fruit, a jelly sandwich, cookies, and a sugar drink.

Question: **How long before game time should the pre-game meal be eaten to allow for digestion to take place?**

Answer: A three-hour time period is sufficient for most athletes.

Question: **Should liquid formula diets be served as a pre-game meal?**

Answer: The liquid formula drinks aren't recommended as a substitute for whole food. They can, however, be used as a supplemental feeding for such events as swimming or track and field when meals are difficult to schedule. Be sure that *each* athlete likes the kind to be used as it could be objectionable to some.

Question: **What about the carbohydrate-loading diets I've read about? Should any female athletes be using it?**

Answer: Even though there are some risks involved in the carbohydrate-loading diet (such as nausea and diarrhea), some long-distance runners may want to try it. If they do, they should do so under advice from physicians and trainers who are experienced in the technique. *Be sure to remember:* most athletic events are of such short duration that no benefit would be obtained from carbohydrate loading. Only continuous activities that last at least 45 minutes (not sports that require stopping and starting), would be benefitted. (See chapter 11 for details on carbohydrate loading.)

Question: **Why does carbohydrate loading work?**

Answer: Because high-carbohydrate diets give the best energy yield per liter of oxygen compared to high-fat, high-protein, and normal-mixed diets. Plus, when carbohydrate loading is practiced properly, glycogen stores in the working muscles are increased. The importance of a high initial level of muscle glycogen is that it enables the athlete who competes in an endurance-type event to maintain her optimal pace for an extended period of time.

Question: **Do female athletes need protein pills?**

Answer: No with a capitol "N". Studies have shown that if female athletes get anything at all out of their diet, they get *more than enough protein.*

Question: **How much protein should a female athlete be eating each day?**

Answer: Since protein is measured in grams, we must understand what a gram is. A gram is the basic unit of weight in the metric system, and is equal to about 1/28 of an ounce. There are 454 grams in a pound. Following this system, food-composition tables list protein in grams. For example: 8 ounces of milk contain 9 grams of protein, a large egg has 6 grams, and a 6-ounce steak has 48 grams. Be sure and examine food-composition tables for complete listings.

Getting back to the question, nutritionists have devised a simple rule of thumb to determine adequate protein levels for female athletes. They recommend *no more* than 0.8 grams of protein, daily, for each kilogram of bodyweight . . . or .39 grams of protein for each pound of bodyweight. You can determine your athletes needs by multiplying their weight in pounds by .39.

Question: **How can diet be used in combating heat stroke?**
Answer: Coaches should urge their athletes to drink liberal amounts of liquids before, during, and after practice sessions, and *salt* on foods. During hot weather, all athletes should be weighed before and after practice. Body-weight loss is probably the easiest way to measure heat acclimatization. If there is more than a 5 percent weight loss, the athlete should be watched carefully and encouraged to drink saline solution.

Question: **Which is better, salt tablets or saline solution, for conditioning to heat?**
Answer: Saline solution (salted water) is more readily available to meet the need of the body. In excessive sweating, water is always lost more than salt, and fluid replacement is essential. Furthermore, salt tablets may cause irritation to the stomach lining or be passed completely undissolved.

Question: **Tell me more about this saline solution. How is it made?**
Answer: A simple formula for a saline solution that costs about 15 cents a gallon is as follows:
1 gallon water,
1 tablespoon iodized salt,
3 tablespoons sugar,
1 package of Kool-Aid for color,
Ice to chill.

Question: **How much and when should saline solution be given?**
Answer: Each athlete should be given at least 10 to 20 ounces (1-3 glasses) per hour. Once again, athletes should be encouraged to drink before, during, and after practice. Once they become accustomed to the heat, a liberal use of *water* and *salt on food* is sufficient.

Question: **It's so hard to keep my girls away from the drive-in hamburger places. How "bad" are the foods they serve for athletes?**

Answer: I know some coaches are going to cringe when I say this, but there is nothing wrong with properly prepared hamburgers, french fries, and milk shakes or malts. Dr. Laurence Finberg of the Albert Einstein College of Medicine analyzed the food of three major fast-food chains and found that a quarter-pound hamburger, order of fries, and a milk shake — consumed several times a day — has nearly all the nutrients needed by growing adolescents, including athletes. For those of you considering eating hamburgers three times a day for several weeks, Dr. Finberg does recommend liver once a week and occasional vegetables.

Question: **What do you recommend for a girl who needs to lose weight?**

Answer: Actually the words *losing weight* are misleading since an athlete can (and many of them do) lose weight without losing fat. Female athletes need as much muscle as they can get, but they would perform much better with a reduced percentage of body fat.

In order to reduce body fat, the body must be forced to burn its own fat as a source of energy. An athlete who consumes 500 calories less a day than her maintenance level will require her body to burn one pound of fat a week (3,500 calories in a pound of fat) as a source of energy. And this 500 calories a day reduction should come from no *one* food group, but from all food groups. In other words, smaller servings should be eaten.

A girl who loses over two pounds of body weight a week on a "crash diet" of some sort can be assured that most of this weight will be from her muscles and organs, not her fat stores. Anything more than a two pound weight loss a week is dangerous. Stick to a well-balanced, lower calorie diet for losing fat.

Question: **What about gaining weight?**

Answer: Once again, gaining weight is one thing, while gaining muscle is totally different. I'm assuming that you want to gain muscle, not fat, since fat contributes nothing to athletic performance.

A pound of muscle contains only 600 calories (and a lot of water), but eating an extra 600 calories won't make any difference as far as building muscle is concerned, *unless you have stimulated muscular growth beforehand.* Muscular growth is stimulated best by a program of progressive resistance exercise performed in a high-intensity fashion.

Most women, because of hormone differences, cannot develop large muscles . . . at least not to the extent that men can. But they *can* significantly *strengthen* their muscles with proper exercise.

Question: **Are there any guidelines that you could give me for developing a strength-building program for female athletes?**

Answer: If you can get a copy of the March-April 1975 issue of *Woman Coach,* do so. I've written a comprehensive article, with illustrations, on this very subject.

Without attempting to become involved in a lengthy discussion, the rules for this type of training can be summarized very briefly:

1. Use as many *full-range* movements as possible to insure development of the entire length of the involved muscles, and to increase flexibility.

2. Perform all repetitions in a rather *slow fashion* (accentuating the lowering portion of the movement) and avoid all throwing or jerking movements.

3. Continue each exercise to a point of *momentary muscular failure,* which point should be reached after 8-12 repetitions working against as much resistance as possible.

4. When 12 repetitions can be performed in good form, add 5 pounds the next training session and try to perform at least 8 repetitions.

5. The entire workout should consist of no more than 12 exercise (4-6 for the lower body and 6-8 for the upper body); perform only *one set* of each exercise.

6. Best results occur when there are at least 48 hours and not more than 96 hours between strength-training sessions.

No major differences exist between the way men and women athletes should train for strength. Women particularly need to learn that it's the *intensity* of the exercises that builds strength: *the higher the intensity, the better the muscles are stimulated.* No amount of light, calisthenic-type movements will build much in the way of strength. Proper strength training must be *hard, brief,* and *progressive.*

161

Question: **Can you list some specific exercises for women interested in building strength?**

Answer: Women actually have more to gain from strength training than men, because most of the time strength is the weakest link in the physical make-up of a woman. A basic strength-training program for the major muscles of the body utilizing Nautilus exercise machines or barbells would look something like this:

Nautilus Machines	**Barbell Exercises**
1. Hip and Back	1. Squat
2. Compound Leg	2. Pullover
3. Leg Curl	3. Stiff-legged deadlift
4. Pullover Torso-Arm	4. Press
5. Double Shoulder	5. Curl
6. Neck and Shoulder	6. Bench press
7. Double Chest	7. Sit-up

Question: **There used to be a belief that milk caused "cottonmouth." Is this still true?**

Answer: There is no scientific evidence that "cottonmouth" is caused by milk. "Cottonmouth" is usually a result of tension, and tension causes the salivary glands to decrease the flow of saliva. As a result, the mouth becomes dry and feels fuzzy. Water, ice, soft drinks, and chewing gum are effective in combating this condition.

Question: **Should vitamins and other food supplements be routinely given to female athletes?**

Answer: No! A balanced diet made up of the previously described four food groups will provide all the nutrients needed by most athletes.

If taking vitamin pills would truly make the difference between winning and losing, Billie Jean King would have never been able to defeat Bobby Riggs. Riggs was taking 300 to 400 nutrient pills a day in preparation for the so-called "Battle of the Sexes" or "Tennis Match of the Century." His advisor, Rheo H. Blair, a Hollywood "health food" advocate and pseudo-nutritionist, was certain Riggs would be unbeatable after this *supercharged, pill-popping program* had been initiated. The millions of Americans who followed the match should now know better. Consuming such overloads of nutrients is certainly not needed; plus, they can lead to dangerous complications.

For example, there's the case of a 4-year old boy in Kansas who took a whole bottle of 40 children's vitamins at once. He spent the following two days in intensive care with vitamin A and iron poisoning. His experience was added to the statistics compiled by the National Clearinghouse for Poison Control Centers which reveal that 4,000 cases of vitamin poisonings are reported each year.

Question: **I've heard vitamin E taken in large doses will improve stamina. Should my girls be taking it?**

Answer: Vitamin E is a necessary nutrient, but taking large amounts of it in capsule form will not improve an athlete's stamina. This is just another of the many myths that surround the athletic world.

Question: **What about vitamin C tablets? Won't they help prevent colds?**

Answer: The value of vitamin C in preventing colds is still controversial. Most nutrition experts note, however, that the massive doses recommended (up to 5,000 mg. in pill form a day) can cause diarrhea, excessive urination, and kidney and bladder stones. And they question its value in preventing colds.

Until more conclusive evidence is available, the athlete needn't consume more than the normal daily vitamin C requirement . . . which is easily obtainable from four servings of fruits and vegetables.

Question: **I've read where nutritionists say many women are deficient in iron. Should iron pills be available to women athletes?**

Answer: Many women are deficient in iron. If an athlete shows signs of unusual fatigue about mid-season, she should be sent to a physician to have her hemoglobin checked. If the iron in her blood is low, the physician will prescribe the appropriate iron supplement.

Since the body can only absorb about one-tenth of the iron consumed, females need 18 mg. of iron a day to extract from 1 mg. to 2 mg. Good sources of iron are meats, enriched bread and cereal, leafy vegetables, and dried fruits. Dried apricots and raisins are excellent iron-rich snacks for athletes. Wash it down with orange juice because vitamin C is necessary in the intestinal tract for the absorption of iron.

Question: **Are there any other nutritional-related problems that are specific to female athletes that you haven't discussed?**

Answer: Perhaps something should be said about menstruation. Normal menstruation involves a small loss of iron and protein, both of which will be easily replaced by good nutrition throughout the month. Approximately 5 percent of female athletes will have excessive menstrual flows. If you are in this group, be sure to increase your consumption of iron-rich foods, especially before and during your period.

Another related problem concerns the nutritional effects of birth control pills. Coaches and athletes should be aware that oral contraceptive drugs may cause certain nutrient deficiencies, such as: vitamin C, folic acid, and an essential amino acid — tryptophan. A well-balanced diet is especially important to women athletes taking these drugs.

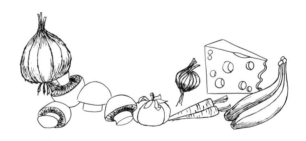

11

How to Eat
Like a Champion

FROM THE preceding chapters, it can be seen that there is little evidence that athletes have special nutritional requirements. However, certain considerations and recommendations have been found useful by competent physicians, trainers, coaches, and athletes. Such topics as patterns of eating, composition of meals, pre-game meals, losing body fat, and gaining weight warrant further discussion.

PATTERNS OF EATING AND PERFORMANCE

The influence of the number and spacing of meals has been studied in relation to the effect upon physical performance. Several scientists have found that frequent meals led to higher levels of performance and they maintain that total work output could be increased by using a pattern of five meals per day. Drs. Jean Mayer and Beverly Bullen of Harvard University in a 1960 edition of *Physiological Review,* have also concluded that frequent, moderate-sized meals may produce a maximum efficiency from the psychological standpoint. Long intervals between meals tend to have unfavorable effects. However, they conclude that with the possible exception of breakfast, the ingestion of food is not followed by a great increase in productivity or improvement in physical performance.

To the athlete, breakfast should be one of the most important meals, yet it is often neglected. A scientist with the U.S. Department of Agriculture studied 3,500 high school students in

Massachusetts and found that 11 percent of the boys and 19 percent of the girls had a poor breakfast or skipped it altogether. It was also found that when breakfast was skipped, the students took longer to make decisions, were less steady, and their work output was less. Therefore, it is recommended that the growing athlete eat a hearty breakfast and consume from three to five moderate sized and balanced meals per day to produce maximum efficiency during athletic performance.

COMPOSITION OF MEALS AND PERFORMANCE (CARBOHYDRATE LOADING)

In physical activity or athletic events lasting less than 45 minutes, the usual supply of stored energy is sufficient to supply the energy need. Under such conditions the diet is of minor importance. However, when an athlete must work in heavy physical activity for periods exceeding 45 minutes, special training and diet procedures are required. A carbohydrate-rich diet is recommended for several days prior to competition. But, it is not advisable to live on a high-carbohydrate diet regularly, since this would condition the metabolic processes to a high utilization of carbohydrate fuel rather than fats.

Therefore, nutritional scientists recommend that athletes involved in sporting events exceeding 45 minutes should: (1) deplete their glycogen stores by exercising to exhaustion the same muscles that will be used in competition . . . this should be done about one week prior to competition; (2) the diet should be almost exclusively fat and protein for the next days; (3) more exercise should be done three days prior to competition to ensure that absence of glycogen; (4) then the athlete should add large quantities of carbohydrates to his diet for the next days, or until the competition begins. (Athletes involved in prolonged competition should also consume weak sugar drinks during and between matches.)

The following three phases show specific guidelines that can be adhered to prior to an important game, contest, or tournament, which for example, begins on a Saturday morning.

	DAYS BEFORE TOURNAMENT	TRAINING	DIET
Phase I	8 days — Friday	Normal	Normal, mixed diet
	7 days — Saturday	Normal	Normal, mixed diet

Phase II	6 days — Sunday	Long workout: 2½-3 hours	High-Protein and fat, low in carbohydrates
	5 days — Monday	Rest	High-protein and fat, low in carbohydrates
	4 days — Tuesday	Light activity	High-protein and fat, low in carbohydrates
Phase III	3 days — Wednesday	Hard one hour workout to ensure no glycogen left	High-carbohydrates, low in protein and fat
	2 days — Thursday	Rest	High-carbohydrate, low in protein and fat
	1 day — Friday	Rest	High-carbohydrate, low in protein and fat
	Saturday	Competition	High-carbohydrate, low in protein and fat; weak sugar drinks during competition

The following foods are grouped under the headings of high-fat/protein and high-carbohydrate foods:

High-fat/protein foods: Meat, poultry, fish, cheese, eggs, nuts, butter. (It should be noted that outside of gelatin, which is almost pure protein, most protein foods contain high percentages of fat.)

High-carbohydrate foods: Sugar, honey, candy, bread, cereals, cookies, dried fruit, potatoes (not fried), fruit and fruit juices, jams and jellies, spaghetti, rice.

These nutritional guidelines apply only to the six days prior to competition. Diet and activity should be normal at all other times (Phase I). Phase II lasts for three days or 72 hours and is immediately followed by Phase III which lasts for three days. Best results from the program will occur if the dietary recommendations are strictly practiced. And "strict" means that 90 percent of the diet in Phase II should be fat/protein, and 90 percent of the diet should be carbohydrate in Phase III. Also it is recommended that this six or seven-day diet be practiced no more than *once every six weeks*. Complications could exist if it is practiced more frequently. Only a very important competition or tournament would merit such preparation.

PRE-GAME MEALS

The important consideration concerning the composition of meals prior to competition is that they should not interfere with the physical and psychological stresses that surround performance. Several previously discussed factors should be reviewed as guidelines for pre-game meals.

1. *Water and salt balance.* The requirements for water and salt can be met by the ingestion of a salted liquid (saline solution) such as bouillon or prepared "thirst drinks" prior to, during, and after the event. You should be careful not to drink too much liquid in the hour preceding before the contest, as elimination might present some problems during the contest.

2. *Avoidance of bulky foods, highly spiced foods, and proteins.* The necessity for urinary or bowel excretion during athletic performance can be serious or even disabling. End products of excessive protein intake are eliminated by urinary excretion. Therefore a minimum amount of protein should be ingested during the meal preceding the event. Likewise, bulky foods such as lettuce, tomatoes, and cereals, and highly spiced foods should be eliminated on the day of the contest.

3. *Carbohydrate loading.* For endurance events (45 minutes or longer), carbohydrate is a better fuel for the body than fat or protein. Under ideal training and dietary conditions Dr. Per-Olof Astrand recommends the training procedure described previously. Carbohydrate or nutrient content of the actual pre-game meal has not been found to be very important.

4. *Tea, coffee, alcohol, tobacco, drugs.* None of these stimulants can be justified as part of the training program of the athlete who wants to achieve his total potential. There are good reasons why you should avoid the use of such stimulants at all times. Although tea and coffee appear to be harmless to some individuals, they are stimulants and a depressing effect can set in three or four hours later, thus impairing performance. Even small amounts of alcohol may be detrimental to coordination and should be avoided. Tobacco smoking definitely hinders neuromuscular and cardiovascular performance. Drugs have not been perfected to the point that their benefits outweigh their immediate or long-term detrimental side effects.

5. *Feeding during contests.* Some sugar feeding during a long exhausting contest does improve performance (e.g., during distance running, swimming, skiing, or perhaps football and basketball). However, the intake of glucose or dextrose pills, pieces of sugar or honey, tends to draw fluid into the gastrointestinal tract for their digestion and absorption and to dehydrate the organism. Sweetened and salted water with lemon or orange seems to be the acceptable way of feeding the athlete during

contests without running into trouble.

LOSING BODY FAT

Numerous people in the United States are overweight for their height, age, and bone structure. This condition is often said to be the nation's most glaring nutritional fault. The major cause of this condition is physical inactivity. Most overweight people in America are over the age of 30; in fact, it has been estimated that one-third of all people over 30 in the United States are seriously overweight or obese.

A person is generally considered obese if he weighs more than 20 percent above the desirable weight for his age and height. However, obesity actually refers to the amount of excess body fat. In other words, a 220-pound football player should really not be considered obese because he is not "over fat" but "over muscled." Numerous athletes are overweight but not obese. The fact that their bodies contain far greater percentages of muscle than the normal man accounts for this condition.

In addition to physical inactivity and muscle hypertrophy, several other factors contribute to incidence of excess weight . . . the principle one being psychological. For various reasons many people have developed the habit of using eating as an escape from the pressures and demands of life. These people must be helped to use more constructive or beneficial means of facing their problems. Other factors that account for overweight are hormone metabolic abnormalities, heredity, and environmental factors.

Losing fat requires a certain amount of knowledge or understanding, discipline, and motivation. Motivation to lose fat must be sufficiently strong to carry a person through a period of adjustment to a new calorie intake that may produce hunger but weight loss. All successful diet plans that are designed to bring about safe weight reduction have certain characteristics in common.

1. *Calorie intake must be less than the body's caloric need.* When the diet supplies less energy than your body needs, the body must use its own stored fat as an energy source. This is the basic principle that all sound reducing diets are based. Therefore, the total fat loss to be achieved depends on how much you are over fat. A reasonable goal or rate of fat loss is from 1½ to 2 pounds a week. Since a pound of body fat has an approximate value of 3,500 calories, a daily deficit of 1,000 calories would

result in a 7,000-calorie loss in one week, or about 2 pounds. This would mean cutting a 2,200 calorie diet to about 1,200 calories a day (see Table 11-1). A person could learn to live comfortably and be assured of nutritional adequacy on such a diet.

TABLE 11-1
1200 CALORIE DIET

	Energy Cal.	Prot., gm	Fat, gm	CHO, gm
BREAKFAST				
Orange juice (½ glass)	54	1	tr	14
Egg (1)	77	6	6	tr
Toast, w.w. (1 sl) plus 1 tsp butter	88	2	4	11
Milk, skimmed (1 glass)	87	9	tr	13
(Coffee, if desired, no cream or sugar)	0	0	0	0
	306	18	10	38
LUNCH				
Broiled meat patty (2 oz)	200	13	17	0
Green beans (2/3 c) with 1 tsp butter	51	1	4	4
Celery sticks (1 c)	18	1	tr	4
Apricots (4 medium halves + 2 tbsp syrup) without added sugar	100	1	tr	26
	369	16	21	34
DINNER				
Pot roast of beef (3 oz)	245	22	16	0
Carrots (2/3 c) with 1 tsp butter	62	1	4	6
Head lettuce (1/5 head) with lemon juice	7	1	tr	1
Bread w.w. (1 sl)	55	2	1	11
Milk, skimmed (1 glass)	87	9	tr	13
Pineapple, fresh (2/3 c)	50	tr	tr	13
	506	35	21	44

2. *The diet should be built around familiar and appetizing foods.* The closer the diet meals resemble what you are accustomed to eating, the longer you will be willing to continue a weight-control diet. Familiar foods are like old friends, they're comforting. Care should be taken to make food attractive and tasty, as eating should be a pleasure rather than a chore — even when losing fat.

3. *Meals should be satisfying.* Successful reducing diets must eliminate hunger and be satisfying. Otherwise, the dieter is likely to frequently "break" his diet. One way to accomplish this is to include more low calorie — high fiber foods, to divide the three or more meals evenly as far as calories and nutrients are

Figure 11-2

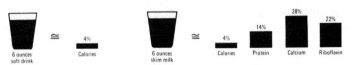

6 ounces soft drink ≅ Calories 4%

6 ounces skim milk ≅ Calories 4% Protein 14% Calcium 28% Riboflavin 22%

Nutrients make the difference: a comparison between equal amounts of skim milk and soft drink (100 percent = the R.D.A. for women 18 to 22 years of age).

concerned — breakfast included, and to take off fat at a reasonable rate or not too rapidly from severe dietary restrictions.

4. *The diet should be adequate nutritionally.* A nutritionally complete diet with less calories can mean improved health and a greater sense of well-being for the overweight person. Empty calories must be kept to a minimum in order for the dieter to succeed. For example, Figure 11-2 shows how two foods of the same amount can furnish about the same number of calories, but different nutrients. Well-balanced diets are still the most important consideration to the dieter.

GAINING WEIGHT

Underweight is not as common in the United States as in some counties. Nevertheless, there are many underweight people in this country who need to gain bodyweight. The cause of the underweight condition must first be established. You can make a good preliminary judgement or learn a lot about yourself by recording your caloric and nutrient intake and calculating your caloric expenditure for a typical day. And be honest — you are trying to learn the truth about yourself!

If you have been spending (using) more than you've been earning (eating) then the cause of your deficit condition (underweight) is obvious. If the cause is not obvious or if you have other symptoms of ill health, you should see a doctor in order to be sure you don't have a subtle disease condition.

The concept that "skinny is beautiful" has actually captured many young people. They just don't think a woman is attractive unless she is 2 to 5 pounds underweight. Many young ladies go on diets, often crash diets (severe dietary restriction) in order to lose weight when in actual fact they would be at or near their ideal bodyweight if they converted their excess body fat to muscle tissue. The most common deficiency among young people in America today is *muscle tone.*

171

Athletes frequently desire to gain weight in hopes that the added poundage will make them bigger and stronger and thus a better performer. Many times extra weight will aid performance, provided it is solid, well-distributed muscle. It is not unusual for motivated athletes to undergo a year or so of progressive resistance exercising along with the proper diet, and actually double the muscular bulk of those muscles directly employed in performing normal physical activities.

Some people appear to be very efficient in the use of their diets or nutrient intake. They seem to store everything they eat, and are always fighting the "battle of the bulge." Other people appear to be very inefficient and can never gain weight.

A number of things can be said about this apparent mystery. First of all, people are different in several ways and it is true the diet that will produce weight gain in one individual may produce weight loss in another.

The people who have an overweight problem often consume more calories than they realize in frequent snack foods they eat throughout the day and night. These people are usually relatively passive or inactive with a slow metabolic rate and just don't burn up many calories.

On the other hand, the people that seem to be plagued by underweight tend to be tense and nervous, have a high metabolic rate and are excessively active often in pointless or wasted activity. These people have a large energy requirement at "rest" or before they participate in a vigorous training program. Such people may find it difficult to consume a diet which provides adequate energy nutrients to satisfy all their requirements.

Several guidelines can be stated that are useful for those desiring to gain bodyweight.

1. *The caloric intake must be equal to or slightly greater than the body's caloric need.* This can be accomplished by eating an extra helping of each food or by eating snacks. Many people have also found that frequent small meals (from 5 to 7) sometimes help them eat more, and at the same time not feel bloated. However as in losing weight, you should not try to overdo this process and be sure that the gain in weight is not merely excess˙ fat but well-distributed muscle tissue.

2. *Exercise may stimulate appetite.* A limited amount of exercise in fresh air may stimulate the appetite and normal elimination without expending large amounts of energy. Also, brief

intense progressive resistance exercise for the larger muscles of the body can be used to promote muscular growth for added bodyweight.

3. *Energy should be conserved when possible.* Living at a rapid pace in an atmosphere of tension with little time for relaxation prevents the efficient utilization of the diet. You should try to slow the tempo of living, get more rest and sleep, and reduce unnecessary physical activity.

4. *Consume a wide variety of foods.* Gaining weight can be boring especially if the same foods are consumed day in and day out. Therefore the meals should be carefully prepared and varied, even to the extent of including rich exotic foods from other countries. Socialization or eating with friends also can stimulate the appetite. Athletes frequently consume high-calorie blender drinks that provide the necessary calories during the intensive training or conditioning phase and are conducive to gaining weight. Such foods as ice cream, milk, fruits, honey, and peanut butter are easily blended to make tasty milk shakes that can be ingested several times a day in addition to the regular meals.

Remember, unless you are grossly underweight, the weight you gain should be in the form of muscle, not fat. And it takes just 600 calories to make a pound of muscle, but only if you've stimulated the growth beforehand with proper exercise.

QUESTIONS AND ANSWERS

Question: **I would like to get as big and strong as I can in the next year. Since I live in a large metropolitan area I have access to different training centers that have all types of exercise equipment, such as barbells, dumbbells, the Universal machine, Isokinetics, the Nautilus machines, etc. Which type of equipment is best?**

Answer: As stated previously in Chapter 4, one requirement for developing muscular strength is high-intensity exercise. And you can use the high-intensity principle with most types of exercise equipment. However, for maximum size and strength increase in the shortest possible time, you must use equipment that provides full-range exercise.

Question: **What is full-range exercise?**
Answer: An exercise is full range only if it provides resistance

throughout the entire movement of the involved body parts. Resistance must be provided in the extended (starting) position, throughout the mid range, and in the contracted (finishing) position. Exercise equipment that lacks any of these three basic requirements is not full range. Barbells, the Universal machine, Isokinetics, and the Nautilus equipment all provide resistance in the mid range of movement, but only the Nautilus exercise equipment provides resistance in both the starting and finishing positions. On the one hand, barbells and Universal can provide resistance in either the starting or the finishing position (depending on the exercise), but never in both. On the other hand, Isokinetic exercises have no resistance in either of these two positions.

Nautilus machines are also superior because they provide rotary movement, direct resistance, variable resistance, and balanced resistance. Therefore, if you have access to Nautilus equipment, be sure and take advantage of it. You'll certainly get faster and better results.

Question: Which exercises will help me in football?

Answer: For football, or any sport, you must first decide which muscle group should be developed and which ones should not. Football happens to be a sport that requires greater-than-average strength in all major muscle groups. (Basketball, tennis, and baseball players would also require overall strength, while golfers, swimmers, and gymnasts would need to concentrate more on their upper body development.)

If Nautilus equipment is available, I recommend using the following machines:

1. Hip and Back Machine
2. Compound Leg Machine
3. Leg Curl Machine
4. Calf raise on Multi-Exercise Machine
5. Pullover Machine
6. Double Shoulder Machine
7. Double Chest Machine
8. Bicep/Tricep Machine
9. Four-Way Neck Machine

The following barbell exercises may be substituted if Nautilus machines aren't available:

1. Squat
2. Calf raise

3. Pullover
4. Bench press
5. Press
6. Curl
7. Stiff-legged deadlift
8. Neck harness

Question: **How often should I train?**
Answer: If you train in a high-intensity fashion, you literally can't stand much exercise. In practice, this means that if you are a beginning trainee you should exercise every other day (e.g. three times per week — Monday, Wednesday, Friday). You should perform one set of each exercise and it should take you no more than 40 minutes, at the most, to complete the routine. Advanced trainees, because they handle much heavier resistance with more intensity, must train even less — only two times per week. Remember, brief workouts two or three times per week are best.

Question: **What about strength training during the season?**
Answer: Many players and teams make the mistake of progressing in their strength training until the season starts, and then they slack off or totally ignore it afterward. As a result, their strength levels decrease with each missed workout. In fact, studies have shown that a high level of strength development shows measurable degeneration after as little as 96 hours of normal activity. Therefore, to maintain or increase muscular strength during the season, you should continue your high-intensity training at least twice a week. If possible, workouts should be performed the day after the game and three days later.

Question: **What determines my muscular potential?**
Answer: Your muscular potential is primarily determined by the *length* of your muscles. Not the length of the bone, but the length of the muscle (contractile tissue) from where the tendon attaches to the muscle at one end to where the tendon attaches to the same muscle at the other end. Muscle lengths or bellies that can be easily measured are the triceps of the arm, the gastrocnemius of the calf, and the forearm.

If two men flex the long head of the tricep (with the arm down

175

by the side) and you measured the length of this muscle, you might find vastly different measurements. For example, the length of the first man's tricep might measure 6 inches while the second man's measured 9 inches. The length of the second man's tricep is 50 percent longer than the first man's tricep. As a result, the second man has the potential to have 2.25 times as much cross sectional area ($1.5 \times 1.5 = 2.25$) and 3.375 as much volume or mass ($1.5 \times 1.5 \times 1.5 = 3.375$) to his tricep. Untrained, both of these men have approximately the same arm size, but with proper training, the second man can have a much stronger and larger muscle.

Thus, the length of a given muscle determines its ultimate size. And the length of a muscle is genetic in nature and not subject to improvement.

Question: **I get out of breath easily. What exercises can I do to build up my wind?**

Answer: Several factors are important in building up your "wind" or cardiovascular fitness. (1) The exercise must be hard enough to get your heart rate up to 140-150 beats a minute. (2) Then you must sustain this heart rate for a minimum of 10-12 minutes. (3) And, such exercise should be repeated 3-4 times a week.

In general, the more of the body's large musculature involved in exercise, the easier it will be to reach a heart rate of 140-150 beats a minute. Bicycling, swimming, and running are good examples of large muscle exercises; much better examples than golf or archery.

In addition, recent research reported by Dr. Jim Peterson of the U.S. Military Academy demonstrated that strength training, properly practiced, can significantly improve cardiovascular fitness. In order to achieve this, the rest periods between exercises must be limited to a few seconds. Done in proper fashion, an athlete can not only improve his muscular strength, but his cardiovascular fitness as well . . . all at the same time.

Question: **In sports such as wrestling, judo, and weightlifting, some athletes frequently lose 10 to 15 pounds in a short period of time to compete in a lower bodyweight class. Is this healthy?**

Answer: "Making weight" as this is called, is often accomplished by undergoing very abnormal dietary practices such as starvation and dehydration (water restriction with excessive perspiration) in order to enter a lower body weight classification in which the athlete doesn't really belong. Such a practice allows the athlete to compete against contestants who are normally lighter than he is. Thus an unfair advantage exists even though weight classifications were designed and established to provide competition on an equitable basis. This situation is not only unethical but it is also unhealthy, and has been condemned by the American Medical Association. There is no healthy, safe way to lose weight this fast. And besides, the weight lost in this manner comes mainly from the lean body mass, not the fat stores.

Question: **After I have lost a prescribed amount of excess body fat, what can I do to maintain my new and more desirable weight?**

Answer: While the answer to this question is simple, it is not easy. New habits of eating and exercise or physical activity have to be learned. That is not easy! New habits are hard to learn and old habits are hard to break for an adult. You need to remember that it took a life time to get you into the shape you're in, so it's going to take a little while to regroove. While it is relatively easy to lose weight, it is much more difficult to maintain one's ideal weight. In fact it is very common for body weight to follow a "yo yo pattern." Such a pattern of gluttony-starvation-gluttony is believed to impose a severe stress on the body. The body prefers constancy or regularity, so much so in fact, that some doctors recommend that if you're not serious about maintaining your ideal body weight, forget it!

Thus, if you are going to vacillate between overconsumption and underconsumption, it might be easier on the body for you to remain overweight or underweight. Of course if one is obese or severely underweight such a conclusion would not hold. The point is you really don't have a choice. Anyone who is concerned about optimum health, especially the athlete whose maximum performance in competition demands he be in perfect shape, must come to grips with achieving the proper balance between caloric intake and caloric expenditure, as well as eating a nutritionally balanced diet.

There are a number of reasons why certain people seem to have more difficulty in maintaining their ideal body weight than others. (These have been discussed earlier in this chapter.)

As far as bodyweight stability is concerned some authorities think that it takes at least one year for the adult body to become completely adjusted to a significantly changed bodyweight, both increased and decreased. Discipline, consistency, and patience seem to be the principle factors that determine success.

Question: **Why does fat tend to accumulate around my waist?**

Answer: There are individual tendencies to develop a high density of fat-storage cells in different body areas. This is an inherited characteristic that cannot be altered. Some people naturally accumulate noticeable fat on their legs and hips, others on their back and neck; but generally speaking, most people (especially after the age of 30) tend to store fat around the waist.

The average male college student has approximately 18 percent of his bodyweight in the form of fat, and the average female college student has about 26 percent. About half of this body fat is right under the skin, and a large portion of the other half is around your inner organs. Most authorities seem to think that for optimum performance, an athlete should have 10 percent or less body fat.

Question: **So, if I want to reduce my percentage of body fat, I should do a lot of sit ups and leg raises. Right?**

Answer: Wrong! Sit ups and leg raises will develop your abdominal muscles, but they will do little or nothing to reduce your percentage of body fat. In order to reduce your percentage of body fat, you have to force your body to burn its own fat as a source of energy. To do this, you must keep your daily caloric intake below your maintenance level. Consuming 1,000 less calories a day than your maintenance level will require your body to burn several pounds of body fat a week as a source of energy. But even then, the fat will come from all over your body, not just one spot.

Question: **You mean it's impossible to spot reduce?**

Answer: Yes, that's right. On a reducing diet, fat is mobilized out of the multiple fat cells all over the body, then carried by the bloodstream to the individual active cells in your body, and burned for energy. Thus, fat stores are withdrawn from your total body fat cells and not from any one isolated location.

Question: **What about the wide variety of spot-reducing gadgets? Do any of them work?**
Answer: No! Not only do they not result in permanent fat loss, but many of these gadgets are dangerous. Let's examine some of the most popular ones:

1. Motorized exercycles. — An exercycle is a motorized bicycle that moves your legs and torso for you. Since the machine is pulling your legs up and down, it is doing the work, not you.

2. Electrical shock. — This machine supposedly makes muscles contract involuntarily through small electric charges. Actually the muscle movements are too small to consume enough energy to cause a noticeable reduction in fat. And doctors believe certain of these machines can be dangerous to the heart and other organs that can respond to electrical stimuli.

3. Vibrating belts. — A mechanical vibrating belt may relax you and make you feel better, but it certainly won't remove the fat. Fat cannot be shaken, tickled, beaten, or stroked from your body.

4. Rubber clothes. — These clothes, which range from belts, shorts, and shirts to full outfits, are supposed to make you "sweat off" the fat and inches. Any weight you lose is simply a result of dehydration, which is quickly replaced when you quench your thirst. And none of the water you lose when you sweat comes from your body fat, since fat contains just a small percentage of water.

5. Sauna wraps. — In this principle, your body (or the specific part you want reduced) is wrapped with tape, which has been soaked in a "secret" solution. You then sit in a sauna bath for 30 minutes, and supposedly the secret solution draws the excess fat from your body. Again, you can't passively sweat fat off your body.

Question: **Are weight reducing drugs safe to use in losing weight?**
Answer: When certain hormonal problems contribute to obesity, drugs or other metabolic stimulants may prove helpful. However, these drugs such as thyroxine are very dangerous and must be carefully prescribed by a physician because they can easily upset the body's delicate hormonal balance. Other drugs that act as appetite depressants such as amphetamines, can

179

produce a feeling of satiety. But people tend to adjust to them after a while or else they become too dependent on the drugs for them to be considered safe or to be recommended. Because of this, most reliable physicians have stopped prescribing metabolic stimulants and appetite depressants to their patients.

Question: **Is fasting an acceptable method of reducing weight?**

Answer: Little harm results when a healthy individual abstains from food for a day or two. The individual may or may not observe a drastic weight loss. If the severe restriction of food or many foods is extended, as it might be for an obese subject, it must be carefully controlled so that all of the nutritional requirements are being met.

Recent research has shown that much of the weight loss associated with extended fasts is not due to the loss of stored fat but rather to the loss of non-fat tissue such as essential enzymes, amino acids, minerals, water, and other cell constituents. Starvation can induce hazardous effects not readily recognized. Forms of gout, arthritis, low blood pressure, and anemia have been reported in some patients after relatively short periods of fasting. Furthermore, there are individuals with certain diseases who should never attempt a starvation regimen.

Shorter periods of fasting (up to 3 days) with free access to water or extended periods of fasting (3 to 7 days) with a low-calorie, high-quality protein source such as 3 glasses of skim milk per day and a multiple vitamin supplement on days 2, 4 and 6 would probably be a safe recommendation for a healthy subject. A more reasonable approach for accomplishing weight reduction consists of a modified diet which includes foods high in nutrients but low in calories.

Question: **Many athletes have used formula diets in their weight reduction programs. Is there some special benefit in their use?**

Answer: Formula diets such as instant (dehydrated) products, which supply approximately 900 calories per day, are useful and safe when used with discretion for the slightly overweight person. There is nothing magic about a daily caloric intake of 900 calories. Apparently it was chosen as the basis for formula diets because most people will lose weight on such a low caloric level.

It would probably be unwise for a very active person or an athlete with a requirement of 3,000 to 4,000 calories per day, to reduce his intake to 900 calories.

Formula diet preparations are especially helpful when used as one of the three meals each day such as the noon meal, if one has to eat it away from home. However, formula diets are not complete, so if they constitute the total intake for prolonged periods (greater than a week), they can produce problems. Formula diets are also an expensive source of nutrients when you consider the ready supply of nutritious foods on today's market. Furthermore, persons will achieve more satisfactory and long-term results if they learn new eating habits that do not rely on special diet preparations for an extended period of time.

There is no substitute for the intelligent and imaginative selection and disciplined intake of food as the procedure for achieving and maintaining one's ideal body weight when it is balanced against a program of regular and vigorous physical activity. Actually the selection of a variety of nutritious foods that provide a caloric intake in balance with the body's need is the only long term program that has sound medical judgment behind it.

Question: **Where can the athlete get sound information on the subjects of food and nutrition?**

Answer: Generally speaking, the place to go for authoritative information is not another athlete, not the "health food" stores, and not the library. Libraries try to carry every book published, especially if it is popular, and do not attempt to exercise judgment on its reliability. Libraries contain many books that are just not valid or accurate in many different areas. Relatively large numbers of books have been written on the subject of food and nutrition by chemists, medical doctors, coaches, physiologists, or people who only hold bachelor's degrees, etc. that are full of misinformation and half-truths.

In this book I have attempted to provide some background material on nutrition as well as the answers to many of the questions athletes and coaches are asking. However, if additional questions or problems arise, I recommend that you consult local or national sources that can provide authoritative information on nutrition and food. Many of the reliable sources provide printed materials, films, exhibits, and consulting or other specialty services. A list of some of these sources follows:

Governmental Agencies

National: U.S. Department of Agriculture, U.S. Department of Health, Education, and Welfare

State and local: State, county, and city health departments, state extension services

Nongovernmental groups, institutions, and agencies

National: Council on Foods and Nutrition of the American Medical Association; Food and Nutrition Board, National Academy of Sciences; professional societies — American Dietetic Association, American Home Economics Association, and the American Institue of Nutrition; and the food industry technical and trade associations.

State and local: Visiting nurses' associations; prenatal and well-baby clinics; Dial-a-Dietitian programs; Red Cross chapters; food and nutrition departments of state agricultural colleges; public health departments of universities and colleges; and community service programs of nutrition committees.

For specific addresses in your area, write the American Medical Association, Council on Foods and Nutrition, 535 N. Dearborn Street,Chicago, Illinois 60610.

Question: **Since there are so many fad books on the market concerning nutrition, health, dieting, etc., is it possible to get an approved list about food?**

Answer: A comprehensive list is available from the Council on Foods and Nutrition, American Medical Association, 535 N. Dearborn Street, Chicago, Illinois 60610. This reference list identifies the authors and categorizes the books as (1) recommended, (2) recommended for special purposes, and (3) not recommended. Most of the references are accompanied by an abstract of a book review that appeared in a nutrition, public health, or medical journal. Although a recently published book may not appear on the list, the author may have written other books of a similar nature that have been reviewed. In this case, the reliability of the latter books could be assumed to be very similar to the earlier books.

Question: **Surely it is true that the athlete requires many more if not different nutrients than the non-athlete, right?**

Answer: There are over 50 nutrients that are required for the building, upkeep, and repair of the human body. With four possible exceptions (calories, water, sodium, and chloride), both the athlete and non-athlete have similar nutritional requirements. Consequently, both the athlete and non-athlete should try to consume a mixed diet composed of a wide variety of foods.

The biggest difference in nutrient requirements between the athlete and the non-athlete concerns energy, especially during training or conditioning. The amount of energy expended by the athlete during hard training depends on the intensity and duration of the workout as well as his physiological condition and the efficiency or skill of performance. In other words, the novice and unconditioned athlete would utilize more energy in playing a game of football than the skilled and conditioned athlete. Within athletics, one could also say that those who participate in endurance-type activities expend the most energy and that the most efficient and desirable source of energy for these activities is carbohydrate foods.

The other three nutrients, water and sodium chloride (salt), are also more important to the athlete or active person than the non-athlete or inactive person. These nutrients would be especially important during vigorous training or activity carried out in a hot and humid environment. The athlete must ingest additional water and salt to replenish the losses that occurs during these periods of profuse sweating.

Question: **My father used to be a college athlete and my mother a cheerleader over 20 years ago. Since that time they have let themselves get overweight and out of shape. How can I help them to lose weight and get back into good physical condition?**

Answer: Your parents are no different from the majority of the people in the USA who are over 30 years of age: overweight and out of shape. The solution for your parents' problem is no different from the solution for people of a younger age with the same problem. However, it will probably be more difficult for them to solve because they have grown accustomed to life as they live it. Their life style, activity patterns, occupational commitments, etc., are all deeply ingrained. On the other hand they should be more rational and aware of the serious clinical results that will begin to develop during the 45 to 65 year age group. The body can cope with a lot of abuse but generally it begins to fight a losing battle sometime after 40 years of age.

The solution that has been promoted in this book for such a problem is not an easy one and therefore it is unpopular and unlike the solutions promoted by the food faddists and others. There is no magic pill or equipment that will do the job. The name of the game or the keys to the real solution are honesty, motivation, balanced diet, and exercise.

The first step in any improvement procedure begins with an honest look at where you are. A thorough physical examination should make your parents aware of their unhealthy condition. The fact that you are concerned about them will also help. Perhaps it would also help to point out that overweight and lack of exercise are two of the major causes of heart disease, which kills more Americans than all other diseases combined.

If your parents will be honest and you can motivate them to make some changes, you can then direct them toward the next two steps: balanced diet and exercise. Authorities agree that the most effective weight reducing program involves both caloric restriction and increased exercise or physical activity. Have your mother and father keep a record of what they eat for several days and calculate an average days caloric intake (see Chapter 3 for details). Next you can help them devise a diet that will enable them to lose approximately two pounds a week. Remember, they will probably need from 1,000 to 1,500 calories per day to provide energy for all their body functions (see 1,200 calorie diet in this chapter).

With respect to a safe and realistic activity program, I would recommend books by Dr. Kenneth Cooper. These books by Dr. Cooper describe the need to restore or maintain optimum function of the circulatory (heart and blood vessels), the respiratory (lungs), and large muscle systems of the body. He describes how much and what kinds of activity are necessary for men and women of all ages. He also compares many different activities so you can find the ones you like.

I would also recommend a program of progressive resistance exercise for the major muscles of the body. Not only will muscles get stronger, but they will become more flexible, especially if you train properly. For additional information on this subject, write to the Nautilus Sports/Medical Industries, DeLand, Florida 32720.

Question: **I've been a winner in athletic competition ever since I can remember. Does this mean I have a better**

chance than others of being successful throughout life?

Answer: If you have been a winner all your life, you probably have a strong, well developed and coordinated body. If you have been a winner in competitions involving many contestants, you probably have had good coaching and have been able to achieve much of your potential. Whether you will be successful in other areas of life, is much more difficult to predict.

There are many factors that have an effect or determine whether an athlete will be a winner. These are not identical for each athletic event, nor are they of the same importance. For example, years of careful coaching may be very important in certain events, such as tennis, and much less important in others such as the shot put.

If successful athletes are unique in any way, it is probably in (1) their superior physical endowment or potential and in (2) their self discipline. In other words, to be successful you have to have the potential and then the desire or means to develop or exploit it.

In general, your maximum achievement in all areas of life requires that you identify and obey the physical-emotional-spiritual laws or requirements that affect the release or achievement of your potential. Those laws or requirements can be listed under the following categories:

1. Physical-Mental Needs
   A. Adequate diet, rest, exercise, and personal hygiene
   B. Mental stimulation or challenge relative to capacity
   C. Learn to make rational decisions
2. Social Needs
   A. Communication with people
   B. Cooperation with people of different backgrounds
3. Emotional-Spiritual Needs
   A. Make a satisfactory adjustment to any set of environmental conditions
   B. Integration of all aspects of life into satisfactory goals and effective means of achieving them
   C. Inner peace, deep joy, and sense of fulfillment

Numerous times the athlete is forced to make difficult decisions. He finds himself in situations where he feels forced into doing things that he finds very difficult to justify or defend rationally. So he falls back on the excuse that the end justifies the means: if it will help him win then it's okay. In fact as the athlete grows and the competition increases, he tends to subvert every decision or action to what will help him win. He may realize some of the complications and dangers of overeating to gain weight or drugs to psych him up for the competition, etc., but at the same time he does want to succeed or win. For many athletes, participation in athletic events or sports has become their entire life and winning is a rich reward for a job well-done. If the choice were between living 80 years cautiously and never tasting victory, or living 50 years of risk and winning, which would you choose?

When this happens, the athlete must realize he has been influenced so much by the pressures to win that he has been trapped. Whereas the trophy or winners' platform was supposed to be a reward for a job well done, it has become the end in itself. Athletes will spend a tremendous amount of time, effort, money, and sacrifice in order to be awarded a $25 trophy and stand on a little box for two minutes.

Is this really wrong? What's wrong with winning? There is nothing wrong with winning unless the price is too high. It was clear at the Munich Olympics that the Russians believed that winning was so important that they bought off many of the judges. Don't let yourself get into the same situation. Don't become so specialized in a single activity that you become "empty" or "void" in other areas. And don't be misled to believe that real fulfillment in life is dependent on scoring the winning touchdown or setting a world record.

What happens after a champion athlete reaches an "over the hill state" or is too old to compete successfully? And what about those competitiors who don't have the genetic potential to be a champion in any sport. Are they automatic failures in life? Probably so if they have not worked on developing their "whole being." On the other hand, the person who has striven for a balance in his physical-mental, social, and emotional-spiritual development (regardless of whether he ever achieved athletic stardom), will be a consistent winner in the game of life.

THE WRAP UP

By carefully studying the preceding chapters, one sees that there are no magic or miracle foods available for the athlete nor are his nutritional requirements unique. Carbohydrates seem to be the preferred energy source, especially for endurance activities, and water and salt are a necessary supplement during vigorous physical activity in hot weather. These are the only nutrients that may be required in extra amounts under certain conditions and that may (to this writer's knowledge) safely improve the physical performance of a healthy athlete. Therefore, the concept that a well-balanced diet is all that athletes require for peak performance is valid except for the several situations or nutrients listed above.

The chances that a diet is nutritionally adequate or well balanced are more certain if it includes a variety of foods. A more specific check on whether a diet is nutritionally adequate is the question, "Does it include adequate amounts of the Basic Four?" The Basic Four, which does not stand for the defensive line of the Dallas Cowboys, refers to one way of categorizing the nutrient content of foods. You should memorize these and learn how to judge the nutritional adequacy of a meal or a diet. They are as follows: (1) meat, fish, eggs, poultry and legumes group; (2) milk and milk products group; (3) fruits and vegetables group; and (4) breads and cereals group. The American Medical Association suggests two or more servings a day of the meat or meat equivalent group; two cups of milk a day for adults and four for children and youth; four or more servings of fruits and vegetables; and four or more servings from the bread group. With this kind of variety and these amounts consumed, as adjusted where appropriate for the increased requirements of hard training or condition, there is a good probability that all of the body's nutritional requirements will be met.

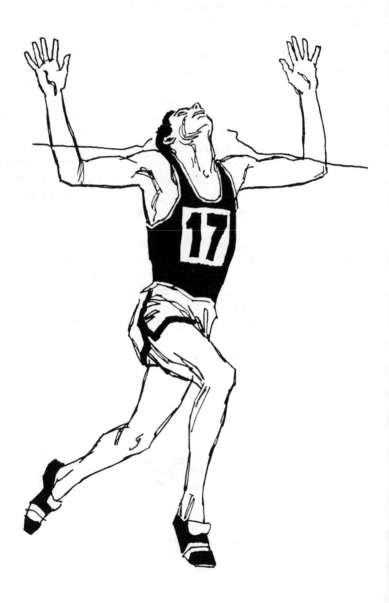

Appendix

Bibliography

Alfin-Slater, Roslyn B., "Vitamin E: Fact and Speculation," *The Medical Aspects of Sports:* 15. American Medical Association, 1974, pp. 22-24.

Allen, M., "How do Athletes Diet?"*Cosmopolitan,* August 1973, pp. 104-106.

Arlin, Marian T., *The Science of Nutrition.* New York, Macmillan & Co., 1972.

Arena, J., "Vitamin Pills and Children," *New York Times,* June 30, 1972, p. 4.

Astrand, Per-Olof, "Diet and Athletic Performance," *Federation Proceedings,* 26:1772-77, 1967.

Astrand, Per-Olof, "The Physiology of Maximal Performance," *Modern Medicine,* 40:50-54, June 26, 1972.

Barrows, C.H., Jr., "Nutrition, Aging, and Genetic Program," *American Journal of Clinical Nutrition,* 25:829-833, 1972.

Bergstrom, J., and Hultman, E., "Muscle Glycogen Systhesis After Exercise: An Enhancing Factor Localized to the Muscle Cells in Man," *Nature,* 210:309-310, 1966.

Bergstrom, J., *et al.,* "Muscle Glycogen and Physical Performance," *Acta Physiologica Scandinavia,* 71:140, 1967.

Bergstrom, J., and Hultman, E., "Nutrition for Maximal Sports Performance," *Journal of the American Medical Association,* 221:999-1006, August 28, 1972.

Bogert, L. Jean, Briggs, George M., and Calloway, Doris Howes, *Nutrition and Physical Fitness.* Philadelphia, W.B. Saunders Co., 1973.

Claney, Margaret S., and Ross, Margaret L., *Nutrition.* Boston, Houghton Mifflin Co., 1966.

Clarkson, E.M. *et al.,* "Slow Sodium: An Oral Slowly Released Sodium Chloride Preparation," *British Medical Journal,* 3:604-607, 1971.

Consolazio, C. Frank, et al., "Effect of Octocosanal, Wheat Germ Oil, and Vitamin E on Performance of Swimming Rats," *Journal of Applied Physiology,* 19:265-267, 1964.

Cooper, Donald L., "Drugs and the Athlete," *Journal of the American Medical Association,* 221:1007-1011, August 28, 1972.

Costill, D.L., Bennett, A., Branam, G., and Eddy, P., "Glucose Ingestion at Rest and During Prolonged Exercise," *Journal of Applied Physiology,* 34:764-769, 1973.

Costill, D.L., and Sparks, K., "Rapid Fluid Replacement Following Thermal Dehydration," *Journal of Applied Physiology,* 34:299-303, 1973.

Costill, D.L., "Muscular Exhaustion During Distance Running," *The Physician and Sportsmedicine,* 2:36-41, October 1974.

Cox, Barry A., and Toohey, Jack V., "Anabolic Steroids and Athletes," *Scholastic Coach,* 40:40, 54, 71, January 1971.

Cureton, Thomas K., "Do Athletes Have Good Nutrition?" *Journal of Physical Education,* 67:22-24, 1961.

Cureton, Thomas K., "Improvements in Physical Fitness Associated With a Course of U.S. Navy Underwater Trainees, With and Without Dietary Supplements," *Research Quarterly,* 34:440-453, 1963.

Darden, Ellington, and Schendel, Harold E., "Dietary Protein and Muscle Building," *Scholastic Coach,* 40:70-76, 1971.

Darden, Ellington, "Olympic Athletes View Vitamins and Victories," *Journal of Home Economics,* 65:8-11, February 1973.

Darden, Ellington, "Are You Eating the Right Foods," *Swimming World,* 15:44-45, February 1974.

Darden, Ellington, "Building Strength and Energy for Sailing," *Sail,* 5:20-28, May 1974.

Darden, Ellington, "The Facts About Protein Foods," *Letterman,* 6:38-40, Sept.-Oct. 1974.

Darden, Ellington, and Ponsonby, David, "Hidden Factors in Soccer Fitness — Part 1," *Soccer World,* 2:16-17, February 1975.

Darden, Ellington, and Ponsonby, David, "Hidden Factors in Soccer Fitness — Part 2," *Soccer World,* 2:22-25, April 1975.

Darden, Ellington, "Strength Training for the Female Athlete," *Woman Coach,* 1:24, 25, 32, March-April 1975.

Deutsch, Ronald M., *The Nuts Among the Berries.* New York, Ballantine Books, 1961.

Fowler, William M., Jr., "The Facts About Ergogenic Aids and Sports Performance." *Journal of Health, Physical Education, and Recreation,* 40:37-42, 1969.

Gilbert, Bill, "Drugs in Sports: Part I," *Sports Illustrated,* 30:64-71, June 23, 1969.

Gilbert, Bill, "Drugs in Sports: Part III," *Sports Illustrated,* 30:30-35, July 7, 1969.

Hedmann, R., "The Available Glycogen in Man and the Connection Between Rate of Oxygen Intake and Carbohydrate Usage," *Acta Physiologica Scandinavia,* 40:305-309, 1957.

Hillsendager, D., and Karpovich, P.V., "Ergogenic Effect of Glycine and Niacin Separately and in Combination," *Research Quarterly,* 35:389-392, 1964.

Hirsch, J., and Knittle, J.L., "Cellularity of Obese and Nonobese Human Adipose Tissue," *Federation Proceedings,* 29:1516-1521, 1970.

Holt, L.E., Jr., *et al,* "The Concept of Protein Stores and its Implications in Diet." *Journal of the American Medical Association,* 181:699-705, 1962.

Ikai, Michio, and Steinhaus, Arthur, "Some Factors Modifying the Expressions of Human Strength," *Journal of Applied Physiology,* 16:157-163, 1961.

Jesse, John, *Strength, Power and Muscular Endurance for Runners and Hurdlers.* Pasadena, The Athletic Press, 1971.

Jesse, John, *Wrestling Physical Conditioning Encyclopedia.* Pasadena, The Athletic Press, 1974.

Jones, Arthur, "High-Intensity Strength-Training," *Scholastic Coach,* 42:46, 47, 117, 118, May 1973.

Jones, Arthur, *Nautilus Training Principles:* Bulletins No. 1 and No. 2, Nautilus Sports/Medical Industries, DeLand, Florida, 1971.

Karpovich, Peter V., *Physiology of Muscular Activity,* Philadelphia, W.B. Saunders, 1965.

Karras, Alex, "Pros' Use of Drugs is Common," *The Miami Herald,* November 23, 1971.

Kozlowski, S., and Saltin, B., "Effect of Sweat Loss on Body Fluids," *Journal of Applied Physiology,* 19:1119-1124, 1964.

Labuza, Theodore P., *The Nutritional Crisis: A Reader,* St. Paul, West Publishing Co., 1975.

Lamb, Lawrence E., *Metabolics: Putting Your Food Energy to Work.* New York, Harper & Row, 1974.

Leaf, A., "Unusual Longevity: The Common Denominators,"

Hospital Practice, 8:75-95, October 1973.

Londeree, Ben, "Pre-event Diet Routine," *Runner's World,* 9:26-29, July 1974.

Martin, Ethel Austin, *Nutrition in Action.* New York, Holt, Rinehart & Winston, Inc., 1971.

Mayer, Jean, and Bullen, Beverly, "Nutrition and Athletic Performance," *Physiological Reviews,* 40:369-397, 1960.

McHenry, E.W., *Basic Nutrition.* Philadelphia, J.B. Lippincott Co., 1963.

Michelsen, Olaf, *Nutrition Science and You.* Washington, D.C., National Science Teachers Association, 1964.

Munro, H.N., "General Aspects of the Regulation of Protein Metabolism by Diet and by Hormones," in Munro, H.N., and Allison, J.B., *Mammalian Protein Metabolism.* New York, Academic Press, 1964.

Nelson, Dale O., "Idiosyncrasies in Training and Diet," *Scholastic Coach,* 30:32-34, May 1961.

Nelson, R.A., and Gastineau, F., "Exceptional Nutrition Needs of the Athlete," *The Medical Aspects of Sports;* 15, American Medical Association, 1974, pp. 19-21.

Nelson, R.A., Anderson, L.F., Gastineau, C.F., *et al.,* "Physiology and Natural History of Obesity," *Journal of the American Medical Association,* 223:627-630, 1973.

Nelson, R.A., Hayles, A.B., Wahner, H.W., "Exercise and Urinary Nitrogen Excretion in Two Chronically Malnourished Subjects," *Mayo Clinic Proceedings,* 48:549-555, 1973.

Nutrition for Athletes: A Handbook for Coaches, Washington, D.C., American Association for Health, Physical Education and Recreation, 1971.

Osius, Theodore G., "Food for the Training Table," *Scholastic Coach,* 30:64-67, October 1960.

Osness, Wayne, "The Effect of the use of Dietary Supplements on High Level Human Performance," *Proceedings of the Scientific Congress of the XXth Olympiad,* Munich, 1972.

Parrish, Bernie, *They Call it a Game.* New York, Dial Press, 1971.

Pauling, Linus, *Vitamin C and the Common Cold.* New York, Bantam Books, 1971.

Peterson, James A., "Total Conditioning: A Case Study," *Athletic Journal,* 56:40-55, September 1975.

Rasch, P.J., and Pierson, W.R., "Effect of a Protein Dietary Supplement on Muscular Strength and Hypertrophy," *American Journal of Clinical Nutrition,* 11:530, 1962.

Ryan, Allan J., "Severe Muscle Cramps After Prolonged Stressful Exercise," *Journal of the American Medical Association,*217:1873, 1971.

Ryan, Allan J., and Allman, Fred L., *Sports Medicine,* New York, Academic Press, 1974.

Schendel, Harold E., *Principles of Nutrition* — Volume 1. Tallahassee, Halmar Associates, 1970.

Scott, Jack, "Athletes Use of Drugs, Common as Sweat Socks — Part I," *St. Petersburg Times,* October 28, 1971.

Sharman, I. M.,*et al.* "The Effects of Vitamin E and Training on Physiological Function and Athletic Performance in Adolescent Swimmers," *British Journal of Nutrition,* 26:265-276, 1971.

Siemann, John W., and Byrd, Ronald, "Vitamin E and Human Work Efficiency," *Florida Journal of Health, Physical Education, and Recreation,* 9:7-8, August 1971.

Starr, Bill, "Behind the Scenes: Anabolics and Amphetamines," *Strength and Health,* 39:54, 55, 68, February 1971.

Taylor, Clara M., and Pye, Orrea, F., *Foundation of Nutrition.* New York, Macmillan & Co., 1966.

"That Man...Pauling!" *Nutrition Today,* 6:16-21, January/February 1971.

Trager, James, "Health Food: Why and Why Not." *Vogue,* January 1971.

Van Handel, Peter, "Drinks for the Road," *Runner's World,* 9:29-31, July 1974.

White, Hilda S., "The Organic Foods Movement," *Food Technology,*26:29-33, April 1972.

Wieder, Robert, "Getting up for the Game," *Women Sports,* 1:54-60, November 1974.

Wilson, Eva D., Fisher, Katherine H., and Fugua, Mary E., *Principles of Nutrition.* New York, John Wiley and Sons, Inc., 1965.

Wohl, Michail G., and Goodhart, Robert S., *Modern Nutrition in Health and Disease.* Philadelphia, Lea and Febiger, 1968.

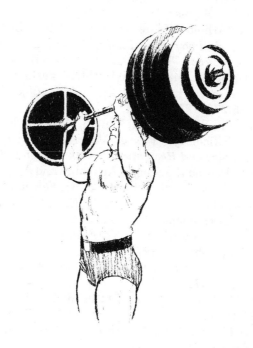

Index

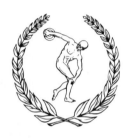

ACKNOWLEDGMENTS

The author owes a special debt of gratitude to Dr. Harold E. Schendel, former Professor in the Food and Nutrition Department of Florida State University. It was Dr. Schendel's concern, knowledge, assistance, and friendship that made _Nutrition and Athletic Performance_ a reality.

I would also like to thank Dr. Robert N. Singer, Professor in the Movement Science Department, Florida State University, for the encouragement he gave me. I am also indebted to the many people who provided their research, information, and data that appear in this book.

My sincere thanks to Donald Duke, publisher of The Athletic Press, for his helpful assistance in guiding an author through the preparation stages on his first book.

NOTES

NOTES

NOTES

NOTES

RECOMMENDATIONS

"Dr. Darden's writing is informative and scholarly, yet simple and concise. In this book he systematically demolishes old wives' tales concerning nutrition and points the way to a national approach. As a physician I recommend the book without reservation. It can be read with benefit by layman, scientist, and physician."

Bernard Sandler, M.D.
Medical Director, Robert W. Johnson
Rehabilitation Institute
John F. Kennedy Medical Center
Edison, New Jersey

"A simple, highly practical critique on the dietary theories and practices designed to improve performance; invaluable for coach, trainer, and athlete."

Scholastic Coach
September 1976 Issue

"The gruelling major league baseball schedule can take a lot out of an athlete. That's why our players are particular about the foods they eat. *Nutrition and Athletic Performance* explains the essentials of good nutrition. I highly recommend this book."

George "Sparky" Anderson — Manager
1976 World Champion Cincinnati Reds

"*Nutrition and Athletic Peformance* written by one of the country's leading authorities on the subject, is 'must' reading for coaches and physical educators. Written in a concise and easily understood manner, it deals with a subject that in the past has been taken too lightly by those who expect to lead athletes up the success ladder."

Glen Wilkes, Ph.D.
Athletic Director and Head Basketball Coach
Stetson University

"After reading this book, I found myself analyzing the amounts and types of foods that I eat daily. I'm now convinced that a nutritionally balanced diet is needed if the body's full potential is to be reached and maintained."

Dave Cowens — All-Pro Basketball Player
Boston Celtics
Most Valuable Player — N.B.A. (1973)

"Athletes, especially football players, should have the desire to learn about their bodies and what training habits make for optimum performance. The contents of this book were meaningful to me . . . particularly the information on pre-game meals, hot weather nutrition, and proper strength training."

Tommy Nobis — All-Pro Linebacker
Atlanta Falcons

"This book is an excellent example of scientific writing for the layman, where a research scientist presents information so clearly and concisely that it can be applied by every interested person."

Thomas K. Bolland, Ph.D.
Post-Doctoral Research Associate
Physics Department
University of Tennessee

"Athletes so often neglect or are misinformed about nutrition. Sure wish I'd read this book in my high-school days."

Dick Butkus
Former All-Pro Middle Linebacker
Chicago Bears

"If you're interested in improving nutritional status as well as athletic performance — you'll find Dr. Darden's book the perfect do-it-yourself kit."

Donna DeVarona
Olympic Champion Swimmer,
1964 Olympic Games
400-meter Individual Medley

"A timely, much-needed book that puts to rest many of the fads and false beliefs that surround food and nutrition. It provides information that can be used by all people . . . from the Olympic champion to the ordinary citizen."

Edward L. Fox, Ph.D.
Professor of Physical Education and
Preventive Medicine
Director, Laboratory of Work Physiology
Ohio State University

"I like this book's approach to nutrition . . . it's a sure winner."

Bob Lundy
Head Trainer
Miami Dolphins

"Sound nutritional research is used as a baseline throughout this book. I'd like every teenager in Georgia to have a copy."

Mary Helen Goodloe, R.D.
Dietary Consultant
Georgia Department of Human Resources

" . . . a book based on scientific and biochemical facts rather than on myths and whims. I'd like to use it in our medical office and Sports Conditioning Clinic as a handbook . . . that can be read and used throughout a person's life, athletic as well as everyday."

Glen A. Almquist, M.D.
Sports Medicine, Orthopedic Surgery
Santa Ana, California

" . . . a much needed book involving an area filled with misconceptions and fallacies. Coaches, trainers, and players can all derive valid information concerning vitamins, proteins, and basic nutrition in a very readable manner."

Larry M. Starr, A.T.C.
Head Trainer
World Champion Cincinnati Reds

"A great book for any one interested in improving performance under stressful or competitive situations."

M.A. Cunningham
Chief, Planning and Support Operations
NASA

"Dr. Darden has made an astute and exceedingly timely contribution to the sports training literature. Anyone interested in athletics will benefit from his training concepts and style of questions and answers."

James D. Key, M.D.
Medical Director, Sports Medicine
Clinic of Dallas
Orthopedic Consultant, Cooper Clinic,
Aerobics Center, Dallas, Texas

"All swimmers and divers should read this book."

Richard Quick
Head Coach, U.S. Swimming Team
1975 World Championships

"Success in an active sport like tennis requires a balance between energy input and energy out put. All the why's and how to's are discussed in Darden's book. Read it!"

Vandy Christie
Tennis Coach
Northwestern University

"At last there's a nutrition book that I can unhesitantly recommend to the thousands of athletes that I have contact with each year."

Pete Brown
Director of Player Personnel
Cincinnati Bengals Football Team

"A clear guide to good eating. I especially liked the chapters on health foods and drugs."

Eddie Lane, A.T.C.
Head Trainer, Dallas Independent
School District

"Being a marathon runner, the kind of food I eat is very important. This book provided sound answers to my many dietary questions. Of course, I liked the special attention Dr. Darden gave to the female athlete."

Gayle Barron
Third Place, 1975 Boston
Marathon, Women's Division

" . . . male or female, young or old, athlete or nonathlete . . . there's something for everyone in this book. I highly recommend it."

Barbara Heller, Ed.D.
Retired Professor of Health
Education
University of California

"Nutrition has always been an important factor in the professional football players' approach to conditioning. It's easy, however, for most athletes to place too much emphasis, or not enough emphasis, on certain foods. You'll find Dr. Darden's book keeps everything in the proper perspective."

Zeke Bratkowski
14-year Pro Quarterback
Pro Football Assistant Coach

"My associations wi[...] at he has combined
the disciplines of phys[...] in the most useful
manner. He is eminently [...]

[...]
Former Chief of Gastroenterology,
Walter Reed Army Institute of Research,
Washington, D.C.

"It's a little harder each year to get in shape. Dr. Darden's book provided me
with some valuable training tips. It can help you, too."

Tony Oliva
American League Batting Champ
1964, 1965, 1971

"As a woman physical educator, I'm frequently asked questions concerning
physical conditioning for females. When questions pertain to diet and nutrition,
one source I recommend is *Nutrition and Athletic Performance* by Ellington
Darden. The chapter on the female athlete is worth more than the price of the
book."

Sue Peterson
Assistant Professor
 Physical Education
Specialist, Women's Self Defense
 and Conditioning
U.S. Military Academy
 at West Point

"The first sensible book I have ever seen published relating to nutrition and
athletic performance."

Albert Schoenfield
Publisher
Swimming World

"This book contains an abundance of information on the best diet and exercise programs for losing and gaining weight."

Tom Laputka
6-year CFL Defensive Tackle
Edmonton Eskimos

"Finally a straightforward, no-nonsense book about nutrition and exercise. No
fad diets, no exercise gimmicks . . . just practical information."

Karo Whitfield
15-year Regional Chairman for
Weightlifting and Physique
Member, Helm's Hall of Fame

"Body builders and weightlifters would save themselves much time and money
if they'd read this book."

Casey Viator
AAU Mr. America, 1971